The Art *and* Science of
Psychopharmacology

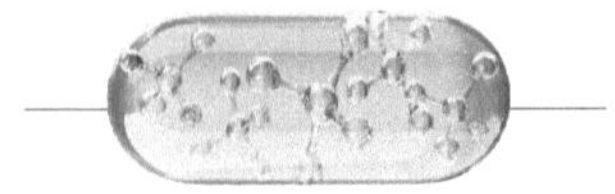

Essential Tools for Treating Anxiety, Depression, Bipolar & Psychosis

Susan Marie, PhD, PMHNP, CARN-AP

Copyright © 2020 Susan Marie

Published by
PESI Publishing & Media
PESI, Inc.
3839 White Ave
Eau Claire, WI 54703

Cover: Amy Rubenzer
Editing: Jenessa Jackson, PhD
Layout: Amy Rubenzer & Bookmasters

ISBN:9781683732778

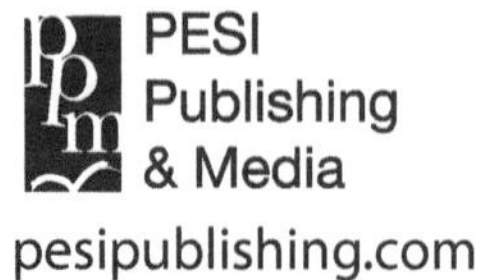

About the Author

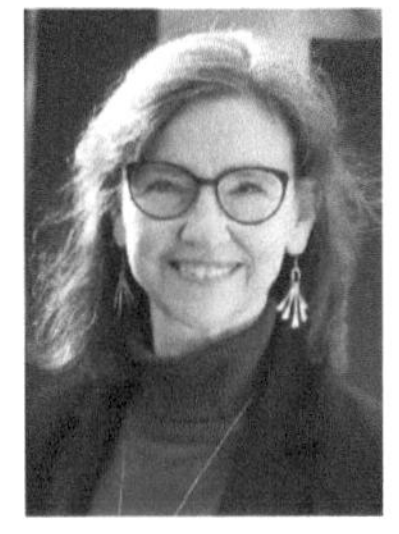 **Susan Marie,** PhD, PMHNP, CARN-AP, has been a licensed psychiatric mental health nurse practitioner for over 35 years working in remote to urban settings in community mental health, addictions, and primary care settings. She earned a bachelors at the College of St. Catherine in St. Paul, Minnesota and masters and doctoral degrees at the University of Utah. She completed and published doctoral research describing life experiences of adults with schizophrenia living in the community. She has been training mental health professionals for over 30 years, and currently teaches seminars nationally to rave reviews in both psychopharmacology and suicide intervention.

Dr. Marie is the Sr. Medical Consultant for Behavioral Health with Central City Concern in Portland, Oregon where she has an independent prescriptive practice treating adults with serious mental illnesses and provides consultation to other psychiatric and primary care providers. She is also an associate professor in the School of Nursing and adjunct faculty in the Dept. of Psychiatry at Oregon Health and Science University.

Susan has two daughters and lives in Portland, Oregon with her partner and tuxedo cat.

Table of Contents

Introduction ix

Chapter

1   *Building the Framework* 1

2   *Treatment of Depression* 13

3   *Treatment of Bipolar Disorders* 41

4   *Treatment of Psychosis and Other Uses of Atypical Antipsychotics* 71

5   *Treatment of Anxiety Disorders* 97

6   *Complementary and Alternative Medication* 119

7   *Going Forward* 125

Appendix A: *Tools for Measuring Change* 127

Appendix B: *Resources for Clients* 129

Appendix C: *Additional Resources for You* 137

References 139

Acknowledgments

What a daunting, wonderful task to thank people who have made this book possible. The material for this book has grown working with mentors and colleagues. Thanks to early mentors Karen Dearing who first spurred me on to graduate school, Craig Brown who worked with radical respect for clients well before recovery was popular, Meredith Alden whose practical aphorisms I still use today, and Bob Greenberg for many, many hours of travel together to and from meetings across remote southern Utah envisioning what behavioral health care could be—and bringing it to reality at Four Corners Mental Health. And a big thanks to Rachel Solotaroff at Central City Concern for years of unabashed confidence in my ability to succeed.

Thank you to many mental health colleagues who expressed interest in this book, and those who attended my PESI seminars and demanded a book! You spurred me on.

Thanks to PESI and amazing editor Karsyn Morse and her team at PESI, and my pre-submission editors Kimberly Hartnett and MariAnne MacGregor. Your invaluable assistance transformed my professional writing into a readable, grammatically correct guide.

And huge thanks to MariAnne for believing in and supporting me carving out the time and energy needed to bring this book into reality and to my daughter Adrienne, for encouraging me to write when this book was only an idea and dream.

My final thanks are to the clients who have shared their experiences and vulnerabilities over the decades with me and for whom this work is dedicated.

Introduction

WHAT IS IN THIS BOOK?

As a mental health provider, you may sometimes find yourself searching for additional resources when it comes to working with clients surrounding the issue of psychiatric medication. For example, you may wonder how you can help clients entertain the possibility of taking medication, or what you can do to increase medication adherence, or how you can help if a client experiences unwanted side effects.

That's where this book comes in: This book provides you with concise, up-to-date, and practical information on psychiatric medications that is based on national and international guidelines and standards. More importantly, it discusses effective strategies for navigating the vulnerabilities and complications of the dynamic and human process of taking psychiatric medication. In addition to information regarding standard dosing, indications, interactions, adverse effects, and the unique concerns and benefits of specific agents, this book provides the information you need to become more knowledgeable, skilled, and an active participant in the process of discussing medication with your clients. With the tools in this book, you will be able to more skillfully help your clients consider the option of effective and safe medication, avoid and respond to adverse side effects, increase adherence, achieve full remission, and ultimately lead more joyful, satisfying lives.

You can use the resources in this book in a variety of ways. If you have specific areas of interest, then you can simply reference that area as noted. For example, perhaps you are interested in learning what is currently considered best practice in the treatment of bipolar disorders. Or, you want to know more about a specific medication to find its common adverse effects and learn when and how to ask your client about those effects to best support them going forward. You can also look up a clinical dilemma, such as finding a client's benzodiazepine dosage and where it falls on a chart of concern, and then research helpful strategies for approaching the client. Wondering how to increase a client's willingness to stay on a medication? This book guides you in the use of metaphors for increasing clients' understanding and motivation. I'll also give you strategies and language to more effectively communicate with prescribers.

Throughout the chapters in this book, you'll find information that addresses specific medications by diagnostic cluster, and I'll also include clinical examples, additional strategies, questions ("Ask Your Client"), and cautions ("Alert Your Client") to help you improve your clients' outcomes with medication. I'll also discuss how to navigate the use of medications with vulnerable populations, such as pregnant women, youth, older adults, and individuals with co-occurring substance use disorders—as well as the challenges of using medications in certain settings.

Ultimately, the tools in this book will allow you to:

1. Help clients better understand how medication works and what to expect

2. Dispel fear and stigma and increase motivation to try medication

3. Understand which diagnoses respond well to medications, including which medications have more robust effectiveness

4. Recognize the adverse effects most likely to cause your client to stop medications

5. Expand your repertoire of questions to better assess adherence and adverse effects

6. Distinguish full remission from response, communicate the dangers of "settling" for response, and know what to do about it

7. Identify which medications can be a resource to decrease suicidality and increase stability in serious mental illnesses

8. Understand when alternative and complementary agents are equally as effective as prescribed medications

9. Recognize concerns surrounding common prescribing patterns

10. Effectively communicate about medications with clients and prescribing colleagues

Who Is This Book For?

The tools in this book are applicable to a wide range of conditions that vary in chronicity and severity, including depression, bipolar disorders, psychosis, and anxiety, as well as other relevant diagnoses. This resource can also be of use across a variety of professional settings, including mental health clinics, substance use disorder treatment agencies, correctional institutions, counseling offices, primary care clinics, and private practices. Regardless of the setting in which it is used, these tools will be of use to any non-prescribing mental health professional, including psychologists, clinical social workers, marriage and family therapists, licensed professional counselors, and those in other related fields.

Given that this book is intended for master's and doctoral level professionals—for whom I assume there is already a foundation of knowledge regarding diagnosis and psychotherapy—this book does not review diagnostic criteria or discuss foundational clinical skills, such as building rapport or motivational interviewing. Instead, what this book *does* do is build on your professional expertise, expanding and deepening your professional ability to help clients through the process of thinking about, deciding to try, and using psychiatric medications—including knowing when and how to discontinue those medications. Although nothing in this book asks you to work beyond your scope of practice, please consider how this material fits within the licensing guidelines of your state and other regulatory body.

Why I Wrote This Book

I wrote this book as America's suicide rate continues to increase while access to psychiatric prescribing professionals goes down. Many clinics have multi-month waiting lists to see a psychiatric prescribing professional. In my own experience as a psychiatric nurse practitioner, I have found that clients lose hope and give up on medications with these kinds of delays. They run out of medications they've been started on, get frustrated with adverse effects, and stop their medication, which results in unnecessarily suffering, including job loss, relationship difficulties, hospitalization, and at times, death by suicide.

These compounding factors—that is, increased client risk combined with decreased access to help—makes it difficult to deliver treatment. And it means that non-prescribing clinicians are a valuable resource when it comes to identifying and advocating on behalf of clients for whom medication is essential and critical. Compared to prescribing professionals, mental health providers frequently see clients for longer and more frequent appointments. However, non-prescribing professionals are often overlooked, if not actively discouraged from talking with their clients about medication. We can and must do better.

By using the tools in this book, you can do just that: You can deepen your existing knowledge regarding psychiatric medication and apply these tools to your day-to-day practice. You can learn the most up-to-date information on clinical decision making, as well as best practices in the field of medicine. With these tools, it is my hope that you will reap joy in your practice as your clients flourish—because they deserve our very best care.

Chapter 1

Building the Framework

As a mental health professional, you play an important role in helping your clients get the most benefit from psychiatric medication. Indeed, there is evidence to suggest that integrating psychotherapy with effective, safe medication results in the most favorable client outcomes (Yatham et al., 2018). For example, medication can help stabilize clients with bipolar disorders or free them from the grip of severe depression, which improves their ability to meaningfully participate in psychotherapy. Similarly, skillful psychotherapy can support clients in getting the most benefit from their medication and can help them develop healthy habits that augment the effectiveness of medication.

So how can you increase the benefits that your clients receive from medication in the context of therapy?

Here are some key strategies for making that happen:

1. Evaluate: Diagnoses or Symptoms?

Treatment begins with connection, assessment, and diagnosis. In the world of psychiatric medication, the issue of differential diagnoses can sometimes make a huge difference in the choice of treatment, and other times not so much. One of the most important diagnostic differences to consider is whether your client has major depressive disorder (and if so, with mixed features or not) or bipolar disorder. These two conditions have different prescribing patterns, and missing the diagnosis can mean many years of continued suffering, disability, and potentially suicide. Similarly, it is very helpful to determine if depression is mild to moderate, or moderate to severe. As you'll learn in Chapter 2, the choice of medication depends on the diagnosis and severity. Your skill and attention to these differences can help improve outcomes and can save lives.

In contrast, the diagnostic difference between schizoaffective disorder and bipolar disorders, while still important, is less vital for determining the optimal medication because both disorders are often prescribed atypical agents that treat psychosis and stabilize mood. Likewise, whether your client has social anxiety disorder or panic disorder matters to your therapy treatment plan, but it's less important in choosing a medication because both disorders tend to respond to the same classes of medication.

The issue of diagnosis is also of concern if you find that your clients are being given medication for the treatment of symptoms (e.g., "anxiety" or insomnia) rather than for a specific diagnosis. Watch carefully. This can be a slippery slope that results in overmedication, often with your client being prescribed multiple medications. When the prescriber is not clear on what diagnosis is being treated, there is an increased tendency to treat symptoms and "try something"—and when that doesn't work, to add another medication to "try something else." Grounding the use of medication within diagnoses is the more effective practice, and this is more likely to happen when you communicate your diagnostic summary to the prescriber.

Compounding the issue of diagnosis versus symptoms is that different diagnoses can have similar symptoms. For example, insomnia can be a symptom of a major depression, or it can be a result of (hypo)mania in bipolar disorders, which makes a dramatic difference in the choice of medication. Likewise, whether your client's anxiety is due to akathisia (a side effect of certain medications), generalized anxiety disorder, or inadequately treated asthma significantly affects the appropriate medication. Again: Treat diagnoses, not symptoms.

2. Knowledge + Choice = Engagement

Many clients have inaccurate impressions about psychiatric medication from social media, movies, and headlines claiming that medications don't work. In order to combat these biases, share what you know about medication and its effectiveness. Talk about which medications are effective for which conditions, which have concerning side effects, and which have the potential for addiction (or not). When you know a medication is effective for your client's concern, talk to them about the specific benefits they are likely to experience. For example, let them know how likely the medication is to improve their sleep, their ability to get to work, their irritability with their partner or child, or their suicidal hopelessness.

In addition, talk about the improvements you've seen with similar clients. How have these clients looked, talked, felt, and acted after taking medication? For clients who exhibit distrust of the medical community, emphasize that these medications are not experimental. Having this discussion is especially important with older African American clients, who may be more wary of taking medication due to past abuses in medical testing. Given that many people are also afraid of getting addicted to psychotropic medications, make sure to talk about which medications are not addictive (when that's true). Above all, make sure to provide clients with ample information and resources. For example, Depression and Bipolar Support Alliance (www.dbsalliance.org) is a good resource for clients interested in learning more about medication for depression and bipolar disorders, and the Massachusetts General Hospital Center for Women's Health (www.womensmentalhealth.org) provides helpful information for clients concerned about the use of psychiatric medication during pregnancy. Each of the following chapters will also provide you with more specific resources to give clients when they would like more information about medication.

Along with providing information, discuss alternatives. For example, when over-the-counter supplements are equally as effective as prescribed medication, review that option. By combining knowledge with choice, you increase your client's engagement in the process and increase the likelihood they will consider medication. This is true for ongoing medication adherence as well. Although you may know which medications are most helpful for your client's concern, it is important to stress that the choice of medication is based on their personal concerns and preferences.

At the same time, do not suggest that your client ask their prescriber for a specific medication simply because *you* think it might be helpful. Doing so is very different from providing information or choices, and it likely goes beyond the scope of your license. In addition, it can cause harm to your client because the prescriber may have to spend time explaining why that medication (or class of medications) is not the best choice of treatment, while not disrupting your relationship with the client. Or, the client may not believe the prescriber and refuse treatment altogether. Both are harmful outcomes.

3. Address Fears and Barriers

Your client is unlikely to volunteer their underlying assumptions, fears, personal experiences, and family history related to medication. However, these factors often represent powerful barriers to seeking psychopharmacological treatment. Asking about your client's concerns and fears—especially their fears—is necessary in order to help them move forward. What have been their previous experiences with medications? What about their friends and family? Do they have fears of "being crazy" or of what other people will think? Stigma is real, and it prevents many clients from trying medication.

In addition, what adverse effects are they worried about? Gaining weight? Being sedated? Bringing these underlying fears and concerns to light increases the likelihood that your client will even consider medication, and it prepares them to talk with a prescriber. Encourage your client to write down their concerns and fears before they meet with the prescriber, as they are otherwise likely to forget important details. In addition, encourage your client to write down any medications they or family members have tried, including those that have worked and those that have resulted in adverse effects.

Once your client begins taking medication, take seriously any and all concerns they have about side effects. It may "only" be dry mouth, but it's often those seemingly small side effects that cause clients to stop medication (see section on Little Problems Matter). Ask them how bad those side effects are. Are they annoying but tolerable? Is the client considering stopping the medication? Perhaps they have already done so. It is okay (and important) for you to ask about your client's experience of medication.

Ask Your Client

- "What experiences have you had with medication in the past?"

- "What have your family members or friends experienced?"

- "Is there anything you've seen in the movies or on TV that worries you?"

- "What about worries that they are addictive?"

- "What side effects are you worried about? For example, sexual problems? Being too sleepy?"

4. Instill Hope and Optimism

A fourth strategy to increase the benefit of medication is to instill a sense of hope and optimism that treatment will work. The human mind exerts a very powerful influence in determining whether or not treatment is perceived as effective. Indeed, this explains the power of the placebo effect: Something that is intended to have no therapeutic value ends up resulting in improvements to the client's condition. The sway of the human mind in determining treatment outcomes is either working for you or against you—but it's always working. Therefore, instilling a sense of hope and optimism regarding the efficacy of psychiatric medication treatment can go a long way.

There are several ways that you can increase your client's confidence in the potential benefit of medication. First, assess how your client currently thinks and feels about medication, which is a process you should have already started by talking about potential barriers. Avoid taking a reassuring approach in this discussion (e.g., "Everything's going to be fine"). Doing so tends to feel dismissive and can increase your client's anxiety about medication. Instead, make comments about what you know—for example, how these medications have been incredibly helpful to clients in similar situations. Let them know that it is entirely reasonable to have hope that this medication will make a real difference in their life. Finishing up your visit, you might say, "You know, it's not unreasonable to think this could make a big difference for you. I've seen it happen with clients pretty often." Or simply, "You have reason to be hopeful." Do not be afraid to express confidence that appropriate medication is safe and effective. You know these medications work for many people. Your client likely does not.

You also help clients trust your judgment regarding psychiatric medication through your professional and office presence. An attitude and atmosphere of competence tells the client they can rely on what you are saying and that your suggestion is worth considering. In addition, be explicit that you will be an active participant in this process. You are not just sending them off to the wild to fend for themselves in the jungle of psychiatric medication. You are interested in their experiences with medication. You welcome their questions, want them to share their experiences, and know how to communicate with their prescriber. By conveying your confidence, accessibility, and empathy with the challenges of taking medication, you encourage clients to be more open and increase their chances of success (Sylvia et al., 2013).

5. Talk Diagnosis (Carefully)

Broaching the topic of medication can bring to the surface client questions about diagnosis that may not have been directly addressed in the context of therapy. This can be uncomfortable, especially if you were taught (either at times, or with certain diagnoses) to avoid accurately diagnosing clients to protect them from discrimination and demoralization—and certainly to avoid talking about those diagnoses. Unfortunately, stigma is associated with some diagnoses. One way to approach this issue is to address symptoms of concern rather than diagnoses per se. Diagnoses are simply professional shorthand for describing a cluster of symptoms that frequently occur together, which facilitates communication.

Medications work for your client, regardless of the label your client gives their experience. Be careful of pushing the issue of diagnosis if your client is resistant to the label of "mental illness." Clients do pursue and take medication while at the same time believing they do not have a mental illness. It is not uncommon for clients to exhibit this cognitive dissonance. Don't challenge it, and don't assume your client needs to believe they have a mental illness in order to take medication.

One way to walk this fine line of educating without challenging their understanding is to ask, "I'm curious, how do you make sense of what you've been struggling with? The trouble with your moods, the irritability, the difficulty sleeping?" Asking these questions is a great starting place because it gives you an opportunity to see the internal language clients use to describe themselves. You can then add to the discussion by going further, such as, "Some medical folks call this cluster of experience bipolar disorders [*or other relevant disorder*]. Have you been told that before?" In sharing this information, you may learn more about their previous experiences with treatment, and you open up access to valuable online resources, which tend to be organized by diagnoses.

In addition, it is highly likely your client's prescriber will talk about diagnosis. Is it better to open this dialogue now instead of your client being offended or surprised when they meet with their prescriber later. You can normalize the experience by emphasizing how this diagnosis doesn't change who they are or what is happening for them. It's just one way of describing their experience, and it doesn't have to correspond with how they would prefer to describe it. That's okay.

6. Address Ambivalence

Some clients are not interested in or not ready to consider medication. In these instances, I find a type of "Columbo" approach helpful, which involves asking questions with a curious, non-judgmental approach—much like Socratic questioning— to help navigate the client's resistance and promote guided discovery. It involves exhibiting genuine interest in the client's thinking with a stance of some confusion. For example, I might say, "You've mentioned you want to be the best mom for your daughters and to do whatever it takes, yet you are not willing to consider medication that is safe and effective. Help me understand what I am missing here." Effectively using this approach requires that you tolerate the client's ambivalence or fears, allow them to be simultaneously fearful of and willing to look into medication, and allow them to say "no thanks" while still holding the door open to talk further in a future visit.

Sharing the limits of our knowledge—what we know and don't know about medication—also increases interest. For example, rather than trying to convince your client medication is a good idea, you can share the following: "Honestly, we don't really know what causes depression, or even exactly how medication works. What we do know is that antidepressants are very effective with severe depression like you are experiencing." Acknowledging what is not known makes medication more approachable.

Giving options also increases interest. When clients are reluctant or fearful to consider medication, I find that offering a menu of choices (e.g., prescription medications, over-the-counter complementary agents with good evidence, therapy, wellness interventions) activates and empowers clients to pursue some avenue of treatment. Often, clients are willing to revisit the menu if they do not feel better in the next month or so.

7. Grieve Loss, Integrate Self

For many clients, there is grief and loss involved in the process of taking medication, or even thinking about taking medication. The deep stigma of mental illness generates deep fears that leave clients wondering, "If I take psychiatric medication, what does that say about me? Who am I then?" It interferes with their very sense of self, and it can result in grief when clients feel they are losing their identity. However, prescribers rarely have time to explore this concern, even though it often interferes with medication compliance and adherence. You can help clients explore these fears by bringing up the issue directly: "If you were to take medication, I'm curious, what would that mean about who you are?" You may want to communicate what you learn to the prescriber; it can be incredibly helpful in increasing the odds for successful treatment.

Once clients begin taking medication, continue to ask about how they integrate this new health behavior into their sense of self. Does it threaten their sense of competence? Of being successful? Capable? Lovable? Or does it feel like they have failed or are "sick"? These questions all provide excellent grist for therapy. Working through these emotions and experiences makes it more likely your client will stay on medication and increases the possibility of better long-term outcomes.

8. Little Problems Matter

It's the annoying side effects that make clients stop their medication, such as dry mouth, feeling sedated during the day, sexual dysfunction, or the feeling of being "not myself." These adverse effects are not uncommon with psychiatric medication, although they often do lessen over time, or actions can be taken to minimize the problem. However, clients usually stop taking their medication before you even have an opportunity to intervene. They tend to not bring up these problems, so it's important you do. Ask whether there are any "little things" about the medication that are irritating or annoying. Are they having thoughts of just stopping it? If so, communicate that with the prescriber. Let the prescriber know both what the problem is and that your client is *thinking about stopping their medication*. That helps get their attention.

Interestingly, prescribers tend to focus on the "serious" side effects of medication—which, of course, are important to assess—but minimize problems without serious consequences or sequelae. However, it is these minor, annoying experiences that cause clients to stop their medication. Dry mouth is a great example. In practice, when your client reports having a dry mouth, prescribers may nod and move on to other questions. They may even make mention of it in their clinical note, but rarely do they ask, "Is it such a problem that you are thinking of just stopping the medication?" Oftentimes, clients think their experiences are unimportant and don't matter, but little annoyances *do* matter.

9. Make Taking Medication a Mindless Process

No one likes taking pills every day. It is a hassle and quite a complex decision-making process. Think about it. The process of taking medication—just one dose—involves remembering to take it in the first place. That means something in your client's environment or daily ritual has to trigger the thought "take my medication." Then, they might have a series of thoughts, such as, "Do I want to take it today? Do I want the hassle of getting up off the couch to go get it? Do I really need it anyway? I'm not sure I really have a mental illness. It probably won't make any difference if I miss one day." Or, they might simply think, "I'll take it later."

When they finally get themselves up, they need to remember where they put the medication. And once they find it, they need to figure out whether they've eaten enough food to take it without making themselves sick (or, conversely, whether they need to take it on an empty stomach). Or, clients may forget they've run out of medication, so they need to stop by the pharmacy first to get a refill. This is assuming the prescriber has called in the refill and the insurance company has covered the prescription. This process happens every single day, and that's assuming the prescriber is dosing it once daily. Twice a day dosing means that same complex ritual happens multiple times a day. We expect clients to go through this ritual when most of us don't even remember to take every single dose of a two-week course of antibiotics. It's amazing our clients stay on medication.

Ask Your Client

Remember, no medication works in the bottle. Regularly ask your clients: "To what degree does taking a daily medication feel like a burden?" and "How do you manage to take your medication all the time? That's hard!" Express kudos and recognition for what it means to stay on medication. It also helps to "get in the weeds" and problem solve how to decrease the hassle of the process.

Setting medication reminders, or asking the pharmacy to pack the pills that need to be taken together, are both good tools that can reduce the hassle of remembering to take daily medication. However, I'm talking about going a step further. I want taking medication to be a process that involves no forethought or decision making. You don't likely debate if you want to put on clothes every day before going out. You just go into autopilot and do it. It might be the same with your morning cup of coffee. The goal is to make taking daily medication a similarly mindless process.

For example, one client I worked with found that putting his medication bottle in his coffee mug helped him remember to take his antidepressant every morning without even thinking about it. Work with your client to find their own version of "bumping into" their medication. This process involves creativity and problem solving, and it's actually fun. My clients seem to enjoy coming up with options, identifying safety concerns, and figuring out a plan given their individual circumstances. And while you're at it, problem solve how to minimize hassles with refills.

Remember, the hassle associated with taking medication is the number one reason people quit, even when they know they need it and their health will suffer. Ask your client to what degree they are already thinking about stopping their medication. Bringing their underlying thoughts and feelings to the surface, and then problem solving through them, is what promotes continued treatment, stability, and health.

10. Talk Their Language

Use the language your client uses when addressing the condition for which they take medication. Doing so will increase the degree to which they feel understood and make it easier for them to accept taking medication. For example, if a client with bipolar disorder talks about "stress," then ask about their experience with their mood stabilizer in terms of stress, not in terms of their diagnosis. Hearing you talk about bipolar disorders may be ego-dystonic and increase ambivalence about taking medication.

Similarly, clients with schizophrenia are particularly sensitive to language given that they have often been subjected to the cultural portrayal of being "crazy."

Clients frequently have more than one understanding or belief about why they take medication, and they may provide several explanations even within one therapy session. This is common. It is also common for clients to see their problem as being related to "stress, not mental illness," while still agreeing to take medication for a diagnosable disorder. Remember, do not assume your client will only take medication if they think they have a mental illness. Clients will be interested in medication if they have some symptom (e.g., insomnia, panic attacks) they want relieved, regardless of whether or not they believe they have a mental illness. That's okay—medications work regardless of your client's personal understanding of what the medication is treating.

11. Never Argue with Success

Sometimes, clients get better with medications that aren't expected to work. And yes, maybe the placebo effect is responsible. And yet the success continues on. Never argue with success. For example, I've seen prolonged remission from depression from an antidepressant dose that, by all expectations, was too low to work. Yet it does. One time, a client told me a certain combination of a low dose antipsychotic and amitriptyline successfully treated her mother's insomnia and worked for her too. I thought I knew better, so I proceeded to follow prescribing guidelines using standard medication choices and dosages, none of which worked.

After months of ineffective treatment, I figuratively threw up my hands and prescribed the low dose combination—which, of course, worked like a charm without any adverse effects. Sometimes, prescribers can be so focused on what "should" work that they miss what does work. When you learn of medications and combinations of medications that have worked for your client or for their biological family, communicate it with the prescriber. That is incredibly useful information. Unless there is some medical reason to discontinue medication (such as dangerous interactions), never argue with success.

12. Measure Change

Interestingly, another way you can augment the effect of medication is to measure changes in your client's symptoms. An intriguing aspect of measuring change is that the *very act of doing so significantly improves outcomes.* Measuring change doubles to triples outcomes across clinical diagnoses. In fact, one study found that measuring change with the use of standardized assessment tools more than doubled the rate at which clients achieved full remission on antidepressants (from 29 percent to 74 percent), and it achieved these results in half the time (10 weeks versus 20 weeks) (Guo et al., 2015). Why is this the case? When you measure change, it provides you with an objective view of the incremental improvements your client is (or is not) making across time. It tends to increase the accuracy of your assessment of distress, which results in more frequent "gentle" medication dose adjustments and greater recognition of adverse effects with more assertive medication changes, all of which are connected to improved outcomes.

There are a variety of readily available, reliable, and valid tools for measuring symptoms, many of which I have included in Appendix A. Use them. Share the results with prescribers. It is impossible to help clients achieve full remission by relying solely on their reports that they feel "better" or still feel "sad." Using this anecdotal information is how clients get *some* benefit but not full remission, and getting to full remission is the goal of psychopharmacological treatment for most disorders. Full remission means your client not only has a happier, calmer life, but it also reduces structural changes in the brain and, for episodic illnesses, significantly decreases the risk of relapse (Pintor et al., 2003).

Another way to measure change is to identify client-specific targets for treatment using the power of imagery. Ask your client to describe what their life would be like if they were in remission. Help them paint a picture of this life, which should include not only relief from their current symptoms, but how their life would look with stability over time. Keep asking about progress toward that vision. Make sure to communicate information regarding this vision, as well as your client's change in scores and any side effects or concerns, to the prescriber. Having this information improves the prescriber's ability to accurately assess progress and affects decisions regarding medication. Because prescribers do not see your client as frequently as you do, they can inadvertently miss side effects or be misled in their assessment of progress by client appearance—such as a client who is having an unusually "good day" or a client who is in crisis on a particular day even though they've actually exhibited overall improvement. Your communication of those measurement tool results helps prevent potential errors.

13. Communicate with Their Prescribing Professional

Finally, communication with prescribing professionals makes a huge difference, but it can be challenging with weeks of phone tag. Some health care systems allow and encourage electronic communication between concurrent providers of care, such as you and your client's prescriber. If you are unable to use electronic communication, consider faxing a handwritten note on your letterhead to the prescriber introducing yourself, and then ask a specific question. Leave the bottom half of the page blank, and ask the prescriber to write their response on that same page and fax it back to you. This process can help avoid medical records—as you are not asking for records, this is point-of-care coordination—and the infamous pile of documents waiting for primary care provider review. Invite them to fax you any questions or concerns they have as well. (Handwrite your fax number in very large numbers on the page!)

If you receive communication from a prescriber, responding immediately reinforces the efficacy and value of communicating. Communicating between treating professionals is authorized by HIPAA, although a release of information is often required by clinics and agencies and is indeed a best practice. Keep release forms available in your office and have the client sign one as you call the prescriber

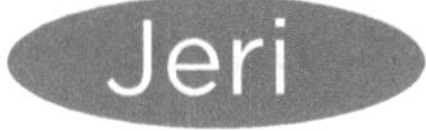

Jeri was a 52-year-old woman who came to see me a number of years ago for a "med check" to see how her medication was working for her severe depression. She presented neatly to our session, with lipstick and curled hair, and maintained good eye contact throughout. She had been taking Zoloft® (sertraline) 50 mg for six weeks. She wasn't having any adverse effects, and the brief headaches and jitteriness she had initially experienced had since gone away. Although she reported she still wasn't sleeping very well and felt "sad," she wasn't tearful or suicidal. In turn, I initially concluded she should continue on her current dose of medication.

However, my clinic had recently started using the Patient Health Questionnaire (PHQ-9), which is a screening tool that measures change in depressive symptoms. So I dutifully gave it to her and was surprised when she scored in the "severe depression" range. When I asked her about the discrepancy between her score and her presentation, she replied, "Oh, what you don't understand is that I got up and took a shower today because I was coming to see you. I haven't been out of bed in weeks." The measurement tool was more accurate than my clinical observation in a quick slice of time, even with significant clinical experience. Yikes.

to get their fax number. Communication increases outcomes for clients. And the prescribers you work with will love you for it.

Conclusion

These 13 strategies provide a framework from which you can get started. In the chapters that follow, I'll include more specific information as it pertains to each diagnostic category so you can build on this framework and increase the benefit your clients receive from medication. At the end of this book, I'll also review some evidence-based complementary and alternative medications for the conditions discussed in this book. Let's dive in.

Chapter 2

Treatment of Depression

Depression afflicts some 300 million people worldwide and is the leading cause of disability according to the World Health Organization (Friedrich, 2017; WHO, 2017). Because it is so prevalent, depression is often considered the "common cold" of mental health. However, this analogy makes it easy to underestimate the suffering and impairment that depression causes. It worsens other medical conditions, results in longer and more frequent hospitalizations, and is associated with poorer prognoses. It increases overall health care costs and—worst of all—quite literally shortens the lives of people who are suffering from it.

Unfortunately, our track record for helping people get well through pharmacological treatment is less than impressive. Approximately one third of people who take antidepressants get fully well, one third get somewhat better, and one third have little to no response to their first antidepressant. Frequently, people require multiple trials and combinations of medications to get fully well. Perseverance is key, as accepting that some improvement is "as good as it gets" leaves clients impaired and increases their risk of experiencing future episodes of depression. It can take some effort to fully treat depression, but it's well worth it.

This chapter focuses on critical information about antidepressant medications, as well as medications used to augment antidepressants when they aren't working. It discusses critical side effects that can result in a client tossing their new prescription into the trash, identifies key questions to ask in order to encourage clients to continue taking medication that *is* working, and gives tips to help clients get better outcomes from medication.

The Bureaucracy of Medication

The Food and Drug Administration (FDA) approves drugs for specific uses ("indications") based on clinical studies ("trials"). These requests for approval primarily come from for-profit pharmaceutical companies that run expensive trials to compile data they can submit to the FDA. Not surprisingly, what motivates drug companies to conduct those expensive trials is potential profit. It is not because the medication will inexpensively decrease suffering and disability. For example, lithium is a natural salt that is extremely inexpensive and has virtually no profit to be made. However, it is not "indicated" for the treatment of depression. Therefore, even though there is an abundance of clinical evidence regarding its efficacy in treating depression, and it is considered a top-of-the-line agent in our guidelines and algorithms, prescribing lithium for depressive episodes is considered "off-label."

When the FDA approves a medication for a specific indication (for example, *preventing* depressive episodes in bipolar disorders), prescribing that medication for a different indication (for example, *treating* depressive episodes in bipolar disorders) is considered off-label prescribing—even though there may be many clinical studies supporting its effectiveness. Off-label prescribing does not necessarily mean that it is "bad" prescribing. It is the responsibility of the prescriber to be knowledgeable of studies and clinical guidelines that address both the effectiveness and cautions against using the medication. Sometimes, drug companies submit medication data from clinical trials to the FDA who then reject the drug because of adverse effects or because it doesn't work well enough. This *denial* of approval is very important. Unfortunately, drug companies do not release this information to the public.

When there have been potentially dangerous adverse effects associated with a drug or class of drugs, the FDA may issue what's called a black box warning. This is exactly what it says—a warning—and it's something to pay attention to. But it is not a contraindication. For example, there is a black box warning on selective serotonin reuptake inhibitors (SSRIs) and other antidepressants for their potential to increase suicidality in youth. Does this mean these medications should never be prescribed? No— it means care must be taken. In this case, it means educating the youth and family members about the possibility of increased risk of suicide and how to watch for suicidality. It means assessing for current suicidality and using evidence-based practices, such as suicide safety planning and cognitive-behavioral therapy (CBT). And it means the prescriber should be starting at an extremely low dose of medication and gradually increasing the dose to prevent akathisia, which is directly correlated with suicidal behaviors. It is a warning to take appropriate measures to prevent harmful, and even life-threatening, outcomes. It does *not* mean the medication should categorically not be prescribed.

Defining Success: Measuring Change in Depression

Drug companies define success as a 50 percent improvement in symptoms. For clients with depression, this "response" clinically correlates with reduced feelings of suicidality and some resumption of functioning (e.g., ability to engage in self-care, go to work, and get the kids to school in the morning). However, it also means clients still feel "off" and lack any sense of passion, joy, or zest for life. As a provider, your goal is to ensure clients achieve full remission—that is, that they regain the capacity to feel joy, whether it involves growing roses in their garden or coaching their child's sports team. When you settle for a partial medication response, your client is predisposed to future episodes of depression, which increases their risk of developing cognitive impairment and dementia later in life (James et al., 2018; Pintor et al., 2013). Always aim for full remission.

Using valid measurement tools is key to helping your clients achieve full remission. For adolescent and adult clients, two options for measuring change are the Patient Health Questionnaire (PHQ-9) and the Quick Inventory of Depressive Symptomatology (QIDS). There is also an adolescent version of the PHQ-9 that is valid for ages 11 to 17. Both versions of the PHQ-9 are publicly available, and the QIDS is available to clinicians who complete a free registration. Both instruments have excellent validity and reliability for screening and measuring change. These tools are available in many languages but do require that the client be literate.

For younger children, I suggest the Center for Epidemiological Studies Depression Scale for Children, which was developed by the National Institute of Mental Health. For older adults age 70 or older, I recommend using the Geriatric Depression Scale, which is easier to complete than the PHQ-9. It does not require that clients think back over the previous two weeks (as is required for the PHQ-9 and others) and requires simple "yes/no" responses. It is also valid for clients with or without mild dementia. Finally, the Edinburgh Postpartum Scale is the tool of choice for mothers (and other parents) in the postpartum period. It is publicly available and focuses less on sleep and somatic concerns than the PHQ-9. A score above 13 is indicative of Postpartum depression (PPD), and a score above 20 indicates medication is needed. Links to these tools are available in Appendix A.

When Prescribed Medication is a Good Choice—or Not

Whether prescription antidepressants are a good treatment choice depends, in part, upon the severity of the illness. Mild to moderate depression responds equally well to over-the-counter "complementary agents" (see Chapter 6) as it does to prescription medication. However, severe depression requires prescription antidepressants, preferably in conjunction with therapy, such as CBT and interpersonal psychotherapy, which both have excellent outcome data. For clients without access to professional psychotherapy, Recovery International® is a mental health self-help organization that offers training in CBT methods and hosts community meetings to help non-professionals use CBT in their everyday life. It also provides access to online materials and telephone support for clients who are unable, or would prefer not, to attend community meetings. And it's free. This and other online resources for depression are provided in Appendix B.

In addition to psychotherapy, there is extremely good outcome data regarding the efficacy of exercise in the treatment of mild to moderate depression. A large meta-analysis of studies totaling over 48,000 participants found that moderate-intensity, regular (several times a week) exercise showed moderate to large effects in treating depression (Wegner et al., 2014). Despite its benefits, it can be difficult to help clients with depression find the motivation to undertake a daily exercise program.

Although adequate sleep, proper nutrition, regular exercise, and psychotherapy are beneficial for anyone with depression, recent guidelines have emphasized the importance of these lifestyle factors for adolescents and young adults (younger than 25) in particular, given the caution required when prescribing antidepressant medication to youth. Because of its risk for increasing suicidality in adolescents and young adults, prescription antidepressants should be reserved for youth with severe depression and as second-line treatment for mild to moderate depression when other interventions have failed (see Vulnerable Populations section on page 34).

The Neurobiology of Antidepressant Medication

Antidepressants work to treat depression by targeting certain neurotransmitters in the brain, such as serotonin, norepinephrine, and dopamine. They do this through a number of different mechanisms. First, a basic review of how this process works: The brain communicates by changing electrical impulses into chemical "messengers" to cross a gap (called a synapse) between nerve cells (or neurons). These chemical messengers (neurotransmitters) carry messages across the gap and deposit the message at the receiving neuron (the post-synaptic receptor site). Receptor sites are specific to individual neurotransmitters. Serotonin, for example, must dock at a serotonin receptor site. After the neurotransmitter releases its message, it is reabsorbed back into the original neuron (a process called reuptake), which is nature's recycling of sorts.

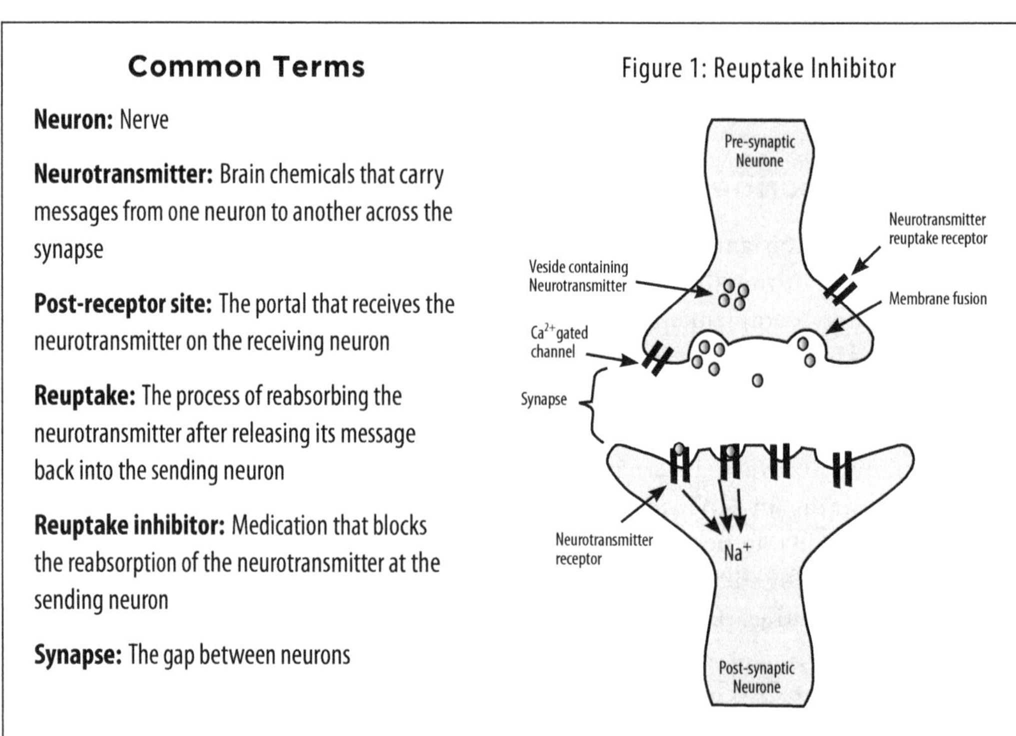

Some antidepressants work by blocking that reuptake. When that happens, the level of available neurotransmitters in the brain increases, which is correlated with decreased depression over the next month or so. Some antidepressants work instead by action at the post-receptor site, still others by a combination of various actions. All of these mechanisms have the result of increasing serotonin, norepinephrine, and/or dopamine. Which neurotransmitters are affected determines the type of side effects your client may experience. No antidepressant is categorically more effective than any other, although individuals frequently respond to one agent or class of agents and not others.

Antidepressants take time to work. Improvement begins within a few weeks, but these medications require a month or longer to fully work. This delay in treatment response is puzzling since neurotransmitter levels increase much sooner than we see improvement. It may be that increasing serotonin and norepinephrine is only the first step in a cascade of actions that eventually improve depression. This complex series of actions builds up a number of neurochemicals over time and increases brain neuroplasticity, which may be what improves depression. This theory is supported by the finding that certain agents, such as ketamine, rapidly increase neuroplasticity and immediately improve depression. It's not known exactly how antidepressants treat depression, but what *is* known is that they work for many people.

How Do Prescribers Decide on an Antidepressant?

Prescribers determine which antidepressant to prescribe their client by considering the following questions:

1. Are there conditions or drug interactions to avoid, or that could be made worse? (Avoid harm)

2. Are there other conditions, in addition to depression, that may benefit from a specific antidepressant as opposed to another (e.g., chronic pain)? (Maximize benefit)

3. Are there other factors that may increase or hinder successful treatment, such as a family history of doing poorly (or very well) on certain medications, insurance prohibitions, dosing challenges, or previous experience with similar agents? (Increase likelihood of success)

Different Types of Antidepressants

Selective Serotonin Reuptake Inhibitors (SSRIs)

Selective serotonin reuptake inhibitors (SSRIs) work by blocking the reuptake of serotonin, which increases the amount of serotonin available in the brain. The term "selective" refers to the fact that these medications only block the reuptake of serotonin; other neurotransmitters are not affected. SSRIs are the most frequently prescribed type of antidepressant and include medications such as Prozac® (fluoxetine), Zoloft (sertraline), Paxil® (paroxetine), Lexapro® (escitalopram), and Celexa® (citalopram). Luvox® (fluvoxamine) is also an SSRI, although it is used primarily for the treatment of obsessive-compulsive disorder (OCD). While Luvox is also effective for depression, the drug company that developed the medication sought FDA approval to market it for OCD rather than competing with other SSRIs coming on the market.*

---

* Note: Brand names will frequently be used in this text for sake of clarity, unless the medication is no longer available or known by that name. However, I am not recommending one particular medication over the others in its class unless I specifically say so.

Some medications, including antidepressants, have slower, more gradual release formulations of the same medication. These longer-release tablets have initials after their names, such as XL (for extended release), CR (for controlled release), SR (for sustained release), and the like. These slower-release formulations do not improve functioning faster or better than standard tablets, but they may be helpful for avoiding side effects, such as decreasing the risk of seizures in the case of Wellbutrin® XL (bupropion) compared to the immediate-release formulation.

SSRI Antidepressants

Brand Name	Generic Name	Starting Dose	Maximum Dose	Comments
Celexa	Citalopram	10-20 mg	40 mg	
Lexapro	Escitalopram	5-10 mg	20+ mg	Can be used at higher doses in practice
Luvox (CR)	Fluvoxamine	50 mg	300 mg	Regular formulation is only generic
Paxil (CR)	Paroxetine	10-20 mg	60 mg	Available in 7.5 mg for hot flashes (as Brisdelle®)
Prozac	Fluoxetine	5-10 mg	80 mg	Available in 20 mg for hot flashes (as Sarafem®)
Zoloft	Sertraline	25-50 mg	200 mg	

Prior to the development of SSRIs in the early 1980s, the only medications for the treatment of depression were the tricyclic antidepressants and the much-lesser-used monoamine oxidase inhibitors (MAOIs). Tricyclics were (and are) very effective for treating depression, but they are also lethal with relatively few pills. Therefore, primary care providers—who are the leading source of care for depression—were reluctant to prescribe these potentially lethal agents without a mental health professional regularly assessing for suicidality. SSRIs on the other hand, are not lethal on overdose, are simpler when it comes to dosing, and have generally fewer and less severe side effects. All of which means that with the advent of SSRIs, primary care providers became much more willing to prescribe antidepressants for clients with depression.

In fact, with the advent of SSRIs, many medical providers and the general public thought depression might be eradicated. However, a significant number of people do not respond to SSRIs or experience intolerable side effects. When that occurs, a medication from a different class is frequently chosen. However, the data shows that trying a second SSRI is equally as effective as switching to a different class of medications. The important thing is to keep trying. Do not give up.

Common Problems and Adverse Effects with SSRIs

One of the most common and troublesome side effects of SSRIs, especially right after starting the medication, is akathisia, which is a distressing, subjective sense of restlessness. It is experienced as jitteriness, restlessness, and difficulty sitting still. Akathisia is similar to how you may feel after drinking too much coffee: restless, fidgety, and perhaps irritable. It begins soon after starting the medication (within hours or days) and can result in a client throwing their prescription bottle in the trash. Although akathisia decreases over time as the body accommodates to the medication, few clients can tolerate the jitteriness long enough to feel that decrease. Adolescents, women, and individuals with anxiety disorders are more vulnerable to this unpleasant side effect.

Fortunately, akathisia can be lessened or prevented by starting the client off with a low dose and then gradually increasing the medication as tolerated. You can also decrease the body's exposure to the medication by having clients break their medication in half. However, some people simply do not tolerate this class of medication at any dosage.

Ask Your Client

When your client is starting an antidepressant, ask about jitteriness. Educate them about this common side effect, communicate to them that it can be easily eliminated, and contact the prescriber when necessary. Simply lowering the dose often helps. When akathisia continues to be a problem, Propranolol® (a blood pressure medication) or benzodiazepines, such as Ativan® (lorazepam), will lessen or eliminate this very uncomfortable adverse effect. By asking, you can potentially prevent abandonment of what could be a successful treatment.

Although clients are commonly concerned about gaining weight when starting an antidepressant, Paxil is the only SSRI with a high likelihood of weight gain. The others tend to cause no or minimal weight gain. Therefore, if your client is experiencing weight gain on an SSRI, that is a concern and a valid reason to contact the prescriber, who will likely change agents. In addition, some 20 percent of people taking SSRIs have excessive sweating. This can be another reason your client may just stop medication, even if it is working. No one likes changing clothes multiple times a day due to excess sweat. This side effect generally requires a change in medication; it doesn't usually just go away with time.

Another common side effect of SSRIs includes sexual dysfunction, which can involve loss of libido or, more commonly, difficulty with orgasm. This side effect waxes and wanes of its own accord. It can be slight and of little consequence to your client, or it can cause them to reject the medication and refuse to try any others. Unfortunately, many clients will simply toss their medication rather than bring up the topic of sexual dysfunction. Be sure to encourage your client to talk about any sexual problems they are having. It is also helpful to alert your client to this potential possibility when they first begin treatment—and to let them know there are things that can help. I let clients know they deserve to be fully well *and* have fun. Putting this on the table helps clients bring up the subject if they experience sexual dysfunction.

Case Example

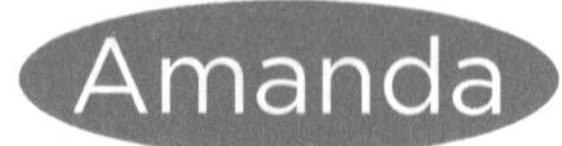

Amanda, who was 34 years old, had suffered through numerous episodes of depression and tried various medications, such as Cymbalta® (duloxetine), Prozac (fluoxetine), and Wellbutrin (bupropion)—all without success. She had gotten somewhat better on a 20 mg dose of Lexapro (escitalopram), and her PHQ-9 score had dropped from 23 (severe depression) down to 17 (moderate depression), but she was still not happy or feeling like herself.

So far, she had tolerated Lexapro better than the other medications, and she hadn't experienced any jitteriness or nausea. I increased her Lexapro to 30 mg, and her PHQ-9 dropped to 8 (mild to no depression) over a few weeks. She was very pleased her higher dose was making a difference, and she started getting involved with her son's school again.

Sooner after, though, she became discouraged because sex had become a problem. She was having difficulty with orgasm and managed this frustration by avoiding sexual intimacy. This lack of sexual contact, in turn, was causing conflict with her partner. She tearfully described stopping Lexapro the past week and was worried her depression would "come back like before."

We reviewed how she could skip a dose the morning of the day she wanted sexual intimacy. That would give the serotonin level in her blood time to drop, and dopamine to increase. She would restart her Lexapro the next morning. She returned a month later and was pleased to report sex was "working again," and her depression remained in remission.

If clients do experience sexual difficulties, there are certain medications that can help improve antidepressant-induced sexual dysfunction, such as BuSpar® (buspirone) and Wellbutrin (bupropion). In my own clinical practice, though, clients often report finding these adjunct medications less than helpful, so I start now with a different strategy that over half of my clients find helpful: the "high-tech" solution of skipping a dose of the antidepressant. Why does that work? SSRIs increase serotonin, but serotonin, in turn, decreases dopamine, which is critical for sexual functioning. Fortunately for our clients, blood levels of serotonin can be lowered (which then increases blood levels of dopamine) by simply skipping a dose of the SSRI, without impacting serotonin levels in the brain or the efficacy of the medication. In clinical practice, clients who are in response or remission are usually able to skip a dose about once weekly without impacting their depression recovery. When this does not work, a pharmacological assist, such as Viagra® or a similar medication, may be helpful for treating sexual dysfunction. This works for women as well as men (Nurnberg et al., 2008).

However, skipping a dose of medication does not work if your client wants sexual activity every day, nor would I recommend it for someone who is still severely depressed when every dose is important. It also shouldn't be used if a client is on Paxil, which has some unique concerns. This SSRI has a very short half-life, which means when your client misses more than one dose, they may get very sick with a flu-like syndrome, feel "electric shocks" up and down their body, and even experience psychotic-like symptoms. The treatment for this is to take a dose of the missed medication. Clients on Paxil may want to keep a two- or three-day dose in an "emergency supply" bottle to prevent running out of medication on a weekend or when they are unable to get a refill for a few days. It may save a trip to the emergency room. Paxil is also not recommended for women thinking about getting pregnant, as it has a higher incidence of adverse impacts on fetal development not seen with other SSRI antidepressants.

SSRI antidepressants are effective 24/7, no matter what time of day they are taken. They work just as well when taken in the morning or at night, and people differ in their experience of activation and sedation. Even though most people find SSRIs activating and prefer taking them in the morning, some people feel sedated for an hour or two after taking their SSRI and prefer to take it at bedtime. Paxil is an exception. It tends to be sedating for most everyone. Educate your client about this. I've had more than a few clients toss their medication because it has made them too tired at work when they take it in the morning. Simply taking the medication at night eliminates the problem.

When it comes to serotonin, it is also possible to get too much of a good thing. Too much serotonin can cause serotonin syndrome, which is an uncommon but dangerous condition characterized by fever, confusion, agitation, sweating, and tremor. A client with serotonin syndrome will look medically ill and need to go to urgent care. It is caused by getting serotonin from multiple sources, such as a high dose of Prozac combined with over-the-counter St. John's wort. It can also possibly occur if a client is taking trazodone for insomnia and a tricyclic antidepressant or tramadol for pain. (Both trazodone and tramadol increase serotonin.) However, high doses of only *one* agent are highly unlikely to cause serotonin syndrome.

Ask Your Client

Be sure to review what supplements your client takes. St. John's wort is contraindicated with prescription SSRI antidepressants. Both increase serotonin and can cause serotonin syndrome, which is a serious, life-threatening condition. Educate clients about this interaction, and let their primary care and other prescribing providers know if they have been taking both.

SSRIs can also cause emotional flattening, in which clients may feel numb or unable to experience any emotions. When this happens, your client may use expressions such as, "I can't feel sad even when I want to" and "I don't feel like myself." The experience of flatness can occur because your client is either (1) not fully treated and only at partial response, as opposed to full remission, or (2) on too much medication. Even slightly decreasing the dose can bring back the full spectrum of emotions while maintaining remission.

Finally, SSRIs are notorious for what is described in the literature as the "Prozac poop-out." For unknown reasons, after your client has been fully in remission for a period of time—weeks, months or even years—depressive symptoms can begin to recur, even though your client is still taking the medication. This experience can be extremely frustrating for your client. Fortunately, a simple increase in dose or switch to another SSRI will return your client to remission. However, depression is so amorphous and pervasive it can be hard to recognize in early relapse or recurrence.

Ask Your Client

Ask your client to describe their typical first symptoms of a depressive episode (e.g., "How do you know when you are first starting to get more depressed? What do you notice first?"). This experience varies widely across individual clients. Note and watch for these early indicators. I also find it helpful to give my clients blank PHQ-9 forms so they can monitor their mood at home and catch depressive symptoms earlier rather than later. Last, educate your client about the possibility of the "Prozac poop-out." Be sure they know it's nothing they are doing wrong! It's about the medication, not them.

Multiple Action Serotonin Antidepressants

Some of the newer antidepressants, Viibryd® (vilazodone) and Trintellix® (vortioxetine), work solely on serotonin but in multiple ways—not just by blocking reuptake—so they are considered multiple action agents. Both Viibryd and Trintellix block the reuptake of serotonin but also increase serotonin through additional, and completely separate, mechanisms of action. They do not rely solely on reuptake inhibition, as the SSRIs do. Trintellix may also have some ability to better improve the "cognitive symptoms" of depression, such as difficulty concentrating. Although these newer antidepressants are equally as effective as other agents, they are more expensive, so they tend not to be first-line agents. Finally, another agent that is also considered a multiple action serotonin antidepressant is trazodone, which was originally marketed in the 1980s under the brand name Desyrel®. When used for depression, it was easy to tell which clients were on it: They were lying flat on their face asleep in the park while their kids ran around unattended. The sedation was problematic.

Multiple Action Serotonin Agents

Brand Name	Generic Name	Starting Dose	Maximum Dose	Comments
Desyrel (was)	Trazodone	50 mg	600 mg	Commonly used only as a sleep aid, not as an antidepressant due to being extremely sedating
Trintellix	Vortioxetine	10 mg	20 mg	Newer agent
Viibryd	Vilazodone	10 mg	40 mg	Newer agent

It's Not All About Serotonin: Adding Norepinephrine

Not all people respond to serotonin, which is why some antidepressants work not only by increasing serotonin, but also by increasing norepinephrine. These so-called "dual action" agents include the serotonin norepinephrine reuptake inhibitors (SNRIs), Remeron® (mirtazapine), and the tricyclic antidepressants. SNRIs work by blocking the reuptake of serotonin and norepinephrine, which increases the availability of both neurotransmitters. SNRIs include Effexor® (venlafaxine), Pristiq® (desvenlafaxine), Cymbalta (duloxetine), and Fetzima® (levomilnacipran).

SNRI Antidepressants

Brand Name	Generic Name	Starting Dose	Maximum Dose	Comments
Cymbalta	Duloxetine	20-30 mg	120 mg	Commonly prescribed for pain
Effexor XR	Venlafaxine, venlafaxlne ER	75 mg	375 mg XR (225 mg ER)	Non-extended release form only in generic

Brand Name	Generic Name	Starting Dose	Maximum Dose	Comments
Fetzima	Levomilnacipran	20 mg	120 mg	Related to Savella®, which is used for fibromyalgia
Pristiq	Desvenlafaxine	25 mg	100 mg	Related to, but no better than, venlafaxine. Doses above 50 mg do not improve response.

Effexor was initially marketed as a promising agent for the treatment of depressive symptoms that had otherwise been unresponsive to other antidepressants. This "treatment-resistant" niche is less promoted today, but many prescribers still turn to Effexor when SSRIs prove ineffective. It has the same side effects as SSRIs, so watch for and ask about akathisia if your client begins taking this medication. In addition, some clients feel tired after taking it, although most find it activating. Effexor can also increase blood pressure, though this effect is uncommon and usually occurs at higher doses (above 150 mg). Ask your client if they've had their blood pressure checked and encourage them to talk to their prescriber if they have increased blood pressure.

Effexor is typically started at 37.5 or 75 mg and titrated every four days or so until it reaches a therapeutic level. Reassure your client that this process is normal and not a sign that the medication is not working. At lower therapeutic doses (such as 75 mg), Effexor acts like an SSRI by working on serotonin. At higher doses (up to 225 mg), it also affects norepinephrine, and at the maximum dose (350-375 mg), it also affects dopamine. There is a wide effective dosage range with this agent. Some clients respond at doses of 75 mg, while others need as much as 375 mg. Increasing the dose gradually decreases the likelihood of nausea and akathisia, and helps determine the lowest dose that is effective.

Effexor has a very short half-life, much like Paxil, which means if your client misses more than one dose, they may also get sick with a similar flu-like syndrome. As with Paxil, clients can treat this syndrome by taking a dose of Effexor—and they can help prevent it by keeping two or three pills in a "emergency supply" bottle.

Pristiq is another type of SNRI that has similar properties to Effexor, as it is also a derivative of venlafaxine. Although Pristiq is purported to result in less sexual dysfunction than other antidepressants, the validity of this claim is debatable. It has the same overall equal efficacy as other antidepressants, but it is more expensive. In contrast to Effexor, it doesn't require titration, which can be an advantage for some clients.

Cymbalta is an SNRI antidepressant with different indications and side effects compared to Effexor and the SSRIs. It is indicated for depression, as well as for structural pain (e.g., arthritis) and neuropathic pain (e.g., fibromyalgia). Therefore, it can serve as a two-for-one agent. Although it can cause significant dizziness during

Case Example

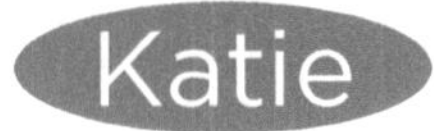

Katie, a 32-year-old mother of a nine-year-old boy, was relieved to have finally gotten her depression under control and, in her words, to have her "life back." She had tried Prozac (fluoxetine) in her 20s, but she didn't like that it made her nervous. Last year, she'd tried Celexa (citalopram), which didn't cause jitteriness but didn't do much to help the depression. During this time, she began suffering from severe depression (PHQ-9 score of 23) with some suicidal ideation, though she denied any planning or intent ("I can't do that. I have to be here for my son").

I started her on a trial of Effexor ER (venlafaxine). After three weeks with no response, I titrated it up to 150 mg daily. She improved, and after another three weeks or so, her PHQ-9 dropped to 17. After three more weeks, her PHQ-9 dropped to a 4 (no depression).

Katie was busy with life. So when she took her son out camping over Labor Day weekend, she didn't think much of forgetting her Effexor. However, by Sunday night, she was feeling sick. By Monday morning, she was feeling "jolts" going up and down her body, was very nauseated and vomiting, and reported "feeling weird." She went to a local emergency room, where they gave her a dose of Effexor. It took a few hours, but she felt back to normal later that day. She came in laughing after the incident and said, "That's the last time I'll ever forget my pills."

the first few weeks, encourage your clients not to give up, as this side effect tends to go away. If clients exhibit actual loss of balance or falling, though, they need to see their provider. In contrast to many other antidepressants, Cymbalta does not cause akathisia, so it may be a very effective agent for clients who have experienced this unpleasant side effect. It also tends to cause less overall activation, so for clients who experience activation as anxiety—and especially for those who also have chronic pain—this medication can be a good choice. There is some evidence that having a current or past alcohol use disorder can increase the risk of liver failure on Cymbalta, though this is rare.

A newer antidepressant, Fetzima (levominacipran), increases mostly norepinephrine, with some effect on serotonin. It is a close relative to Savella (milnacipran), which is indicated for the treatment of fibromyalgia by the FDA. Because it is closely related to Savella, it stands to reason that Fetzima may provide some pain relief in addition to its established antidepressant effect, although it does not have FDA approval for pain. Fetzima is nonetheless used by primary care providers for fibromyalgia and neuropathy. Fetzima requires some titration to prevent nausea that can occur when first taking the medication. Typically, it is started at 20 mg and increased to 40 mg in a week or so, and then increased by 40 mg up to a maximum of 120 mg. Increases above 40 mg are usually done every three to four weeks when the current dose is not effective.

Other Norepinephrine-Based Antidepressants

Remeron is a unique and effective antidepressant that increases both norepinephrine and serotonin but works at the post-synaptic receptor site, so it is not considered an SNRI. Remeron is also different in terms of its typical side effects. For example, it causes significant sedation and is usually taken at bedtime. Compared to many SSRIs and SNRIs, it also rarely causes akathisia and is usually well-tolerated. However, the frequent downside of Remeron is weight gain. For those clients who can tolerate a bit of weight gain, hate the feeling of jitteriness on antidepressants, and are struggling with insomnia, Remeron can be a good choice.

Ask Your Client

Ask your client if they feel sedated on Remeron (mirtazapine). If so, be sure they are taking it at bedtime and not in the morning. Sometimes, pharmacies write out prescriptions for "daily" medications as "in the morning." In addition, ask your client if they have attempted to decrease the dose to decrease the sedation. Let them know the sedation associated with Remeron is inversely related to dose. That is, the lower the dose, the more sedating. Help your client understand when their prescriber increases the dose, it decreases sedation. At high doses (45-60 mg), Remeron can be activating, so clients at the maximum dose (60 mg) may want to take it in the morning.

Wellbutrin (bupropion) is the only antidepressant that has no effect on serotonin. It works as a reuptake inhibitor that builds up norepinephrine and, at higher doses, dopamine. Because Wellbutrin does not impact serotonin, it is sometimes prescribed in conjunction with another SSRI to create a "dual action" antidepressant effect. It also tends to be a more activating antidepressant, so long-acting formulations (ER and XL) should be taken early in the day to prevent insomnia. Due to its activating properties, some environments (e.g., correctional facilities) don't even allow Wellbutrin because taking high doses can create a "buzz." In fact, it can cause a false positive for amphetamines on some urine drug tests.

Wellbutrin can also decrease the seizure threshold, which means it makes the brain more vulnerable to having seizures. This is generally not a problem unless the client has a seizure disorder or a condition that makes them temporarily more vulnerable to seizures—for example, if a client is withdrawing from alcohol or has electrolytic imbalances secondary to anorexia, bulimia, or dehydration. Wellbutrin may also trigger the craving to purge among clients with anorexia or bulimia, so it should not be prescribed to clients with a current or past eating disorder. Wellbutrin is also used as a third- or fourth-line agent for attention-deficit/hyperactivity disorder (ADHD) and is marketed as Zyban® for smoking cessation. Because they contain the same active ingredient (bupropion), clients should absolutely not take Wellbutrin and Zyban together.

Other Antidepressants

Brand Name	Generic Name	Type	Starting Dose	Maximum Dose	Comments
Remeron	Mirtazapine	Norepinephrine/serotonin at post-receptor site	15 mg	60 mg	Commonly used for sleep at a 7.5 mg dose
Wellbutrin	Bupropion (SR, XL)	Norepinephrine/dopamine reuptake inhibitor	75-100 mg	400-450 mg	Risk of seizure increases above 450 mg
Anafranil®	Clomipramine	Tricyclic	25 mg	250 mg	Approved for the treatment of OCD
Elavil® (was)	Amitriptyline	Tricyclic	50 mg	300 mg	Heavy anticholinergic burden
Norpramin®	Desipramine	Tricyclic	50 mg	300 mg	Least sedating of the tricyclics
Pamelor®	Nortriptyline	Tricyclic	25 mg	150 mg	Less anticholinergic burden
Sinequan® (was)	Doxepin	Tricyclic	25 mg	150 mg	At 6 mg dose, it is marked as Silenor® for sleep
Tofranil® (was)	Imipramine	Tricyclic	50 mg	300 mg	

Tricyclic Antidepressants

Tricyclic antidepressants are an older yet highly effective class of antidepressants. They are not used as first-line agents because they are more complicated to prescribe, have some challenging side effects, and are lethal on overdose. These are the agents that (along with the less frequently used MAOIs) were prescribed for depression prior to the development of SSRIs in the 1980s. Tricyclics work on both norepinephrine (primarily) and serotonin (to a lesser degree).

These agents do not usually cause akathisia, so they can be a good choice for clients who do not tolerate the restless and jittery feeling other antidepressants can cause. Because tricyclics tend to be sedating, they can help with the insomnia often associated with depression as well. Doxepin is the most sedating of the tricyclics and is often used as a sleep aid. Like Remeron, the lowest dose is the most sedating. Recently, a very low dose (6 mg) of doxepin was marketed under the brand name Silenor to target sleep maintenance. However, generic doxepin is just as effective as the brand name and is less expensive.

Tricyclics can also be used to treat pain. In fact, your client may be on a low dose tricyclic from their primary care provider for pain. The most common dose for this use is amitriptyline 50 mg at bedtime, though a dose this low is not effective for depression. Anafranil (clomipramine) can also be used to treat the persistent, intrusive thoughts and repetitive behaviors that characterize OCD. Imipramine is another tricyclic that was the first medication approved for treatment of depression in the U.S. It is dosed the same as amitriptyline, but it causes less sedation, dry mouth, blurry vision, and constipation.

A typical daily dose of a tricyclic for depression is 75-150 mg. However, just 1000 mg of these agents (about 10 pills) is lethal, which means your client is receiving a completely lethal prescription every month. Typically, primary care providers prescribe a monthly prescription of tricyclics with 11 refills and never ask about suicidality. Even if providers do ask in June, it means in October when a client becomes profoundly depressed and suicidal, they still get their lethal month's prescription without any review. It goes without saying that giving more than a one-week prescription of a tricyclic to someone who is severely depressed and suicidal is dangerous.

Ask Your Client

Regularly ask about suicidal thoughts for clients who are prescribed tricyclics, even if they do not appear to be suicidal—and even if the medication is prescribed for pain. You cannot tell when someone is suicidal simply by how they look.

Case Example

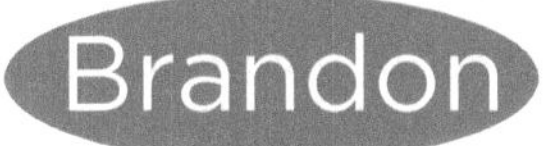

Brandon, 48 years old, was referred to me by his primary care provider. He was suffering with chronic back pain and chronic depression. He'd sworn off taking all antidepressants because they "didn't work" and had caused him significant problems with akathisia. Brandon also had a past opiate use disorder, though he had been clean for several years and was taking suboxone and attending recovery meetings to facilitate his sobriety. In order to treat his chronic pain, his primary care provider had prescribed amitriptyline 50 mg, which he was tolerating, but his PHQ-9 was still 17 (moderate to severe depression). Despite his prolonged depression, he had no suicidal thinking.

After reviewing his history of trying SSRIs and SNRIs, which included Zoloft (sertraline), Celexa (citalopram), Paxil (paroxetine), and Cymbalta (duloxetine), we decided on using a tricyclic antidepressant, since he was already taking one for pain. I switched him to nortriptyline to have less anticholinergic adverse effects, and I gradually increased his dose to 75 mg over a several-week period. He reported tolerating the medication "okay" and was pleased his sleep improved.

After a few more weeks on the medication, he reported his mood was much better (PHQ-9 had dropped to 10) and his pain was also better, both interfering less with his life. He continued to have no suicidality, and over the next few months he started working part-time without any recurrence of his depressive or pain symptoms.

Tricyclics are also complicated by various side effects, albeit different ones than those associated with other antidepressants. Anticholinergic side effects, including dry mouth, blurry vision, and constipation, are the most common. These effects can be alleviated or minimized by drinking plenty of water, using sugarless gum or mints (sugared ones worsen the problem), and taking fiber supplements, such as Metamucil® or FiberCon®. Amitriptyline is the most anticholinergic of the tricyclics, so switching from this medication to nortriptyline can also help, as the latter is equally as effective with only 25 percent of the anticholinergic effects. However, anticholinergic drugs are still linked to increases in cognitive impairment, so tricyclics can be problematic if your client is already struggling with memory problems.

In addition, tricyclics can decrease the seizure threshold and affect cardiac rhythm. This "cardiotoxicity" limits their usefulness in older clients. If your client is over the age of 50 and on a tricyclic antidepressant, they will likely be asked to get an EKG, which is simply to screen for adverse effects and does not necessarily mean they have heart problems. Because of these challenges, tricyclic antidepressants are rarely used as first-line agents for depression. However, they are highly effective and should not be forgotten. If your client has tried "everything," ask if they have ever been on a tricyclic.

Monoamine Oxidase Inhibitors

Monoamine oxidase inhibitors (MAOIs) are a class of antidepressants that are equally as effective as other antidepressants but are rarely used due to their adverse effects, dietary restrictions, and potential drug interactions. This class of medication is typically reserved for treatment-resistant depression. MAOIs absolutely cannot be taken with any other antidepressants and require a "washout" period, which is a period of time after the previous antidepressant has been stopped before the MAOI can be started. In addition, all foods high in tyramine, phenylalanine, and tyrosine must be completely avoided when on these medications to avoid a sudden and dangerous increase in blood pressure. Some examples of foods to avoid are aged cheeses, all cured meats, draft and tap beers, and soy sauce, though this is not an exhaustive list.

Non-Prescription Agents That Treat Depression

There are several over-the-counter, non-prescription wellness supplements that have been proven effective in treating mild to moderate depression, though they are not recommended for severe depression. These include SAM-e (or S-adenosylmethionine), Rhodiola rosea, and St. John's wort. There is some evidence omega-3 fatty acids may also be helpful. More information on these and other complementary and alternative medications is found in Chapter 6.

The Process of Treatment

Conventional wisdom has it that antidepressants take four to six weeks to work and that prescribers should encourage clients to wait it out for results. Actually, very few people who show no response whatsoever at week three or four will suddenly get well at week five or six. These medications result in incremental improvements across time, and you can measure this trajectory by regularly assessing for change with a valid measurement tool. If there is no change by week three or four at a particular dose of medication, it is time to either increase the dose, or if the client is having adverse effects, to change the medication. Indeed, the effectiveness of antidepressant treatment is doubled by advocating incremental, persistent increases in dose until one of three conditions is met: **(1)** The client achieves full remission; **(2)** there are adverse effects and the medication is changed; or **(3)** the maximum dose has been reached, and the medication needs to be changed or augmented (Unützer et al., 2002). Simply put, do not wait six weeks for the same dose to suddenly kick in.

Alert Your Client

Encourage your client to return to see their prescribing provider sooner rather than later when starting a new antidepressant medication. A month is too long, and six weeks is much too long. I aim to see clients every two to three weeks until they get to response (50 percent better) and then see them monthly until they achieve full remission.

Augmentation

Unfortunately, clients often need to try multiple medications, or combinations of medications, in order to achieve full remission. In the past, prescribers believed it was most prudent to keep trying different antidepressants, either by switching agents or switching between classes of agents. However, it is more effective to augment the current antidepressant than to keep trying other antidepressants (Mohamed et al., 2017). Augmentation involves adding a different type of medication to the antidepressant to essentially "supercharge" its effect—and it often works. The most effective augmenting agents are atypical antipsychotics, lithium, and thyroid supplements.

Atypical antipsychotics can serve as an effective adjunct agent when the use of antidepressants alone do not get your client to remission. The required dosage tends to be in the lower range, and the augmentation effect tends to gradually occur over a few weeks. Atypical antipsychotics may be particularly useful for clients with severe depression (a score over 20 on the PHQ-9), one third of whom can experience psychotic-like symptoms. They may begin to hear their name being called, hear footsteps at night, see things out of the corner of their eye, or exhibit increased fear and paranoia. This experience is frightening—both in the moment and over time as they worry they are "going crazy." Make sure to ask about these experiences and reassure your client this is a common symptom with severe depression. Antipsychotic medications will be discussed in greater detail in Chapter 4.

In addition, lithium is the top-line augmentation medication for clients with major depression who also exhibit suicidality. There is no other agent that both treats and prevents suicidality in clients with depression as well as lithium. Lithium cuts rehospitalization rates in half for clients with severe depression compared to those not on lithium (Tiihonen et al., 2017). Frequently, a dose in the lower—but therapeutic—range is effective within a week or two. Lithium will be addressed in more detail in Chapter 3.

Finally, the addition of thyroid supplements is an underutilized gem in treating depression (Zhou et al., 2015). Augmentation with thyroid supplements for the treatment of depression is different than treating hypothyroidism; it involves giving a thyroid supplement to a client who has a normal thyroid level. Some people are unable to translate one form of thyroid hormone (T4) into the form that is useable by the brain (T3), so prescribers will often give Cytomel® (T3) rather than Synthroid® (T4). If your client is receiving a thyroid supplement to augment their depression treatment, it is important they get their blood checked periodically to make sure they are not getting too much thyroid hormone. Although augmenting with thyroid supplements can take a bit longer to work—closer to one month—it often has less adverse effects. Women also seem to respond better to this form of augmentation than men.

Other augmenting agents with some effectiveness include Topamax® (topiramate), Lyrica® (pregabalin), and Deplin® (l-methylfolate). Topamax is an anticonvulsant agent marketed for the treatment of migraines and prevention of seizures, whereas Lyrica is an anticonvulsant used to treat neuropathic pain. Both of these medications may be useful augments in the treatment of depression, although the studies are not as strong as the other augmenting agents discussed here.

Finally, individuals with depression may benefit from augmenting their antidepressant regimen with Deplin, which contains an active form of folate (l-methylfolate) that the brain needs to utilize antidepressants. In order for the body to utilize folate, it needs to convert folic acid (which is inexpensive and readily available) into l-methylfolate. However, up to 70 percent of individuals with depression may have a genetic impairment that interferes with this conversion process (Kelly et al., 2014). In these cases, the evidence for Deplin is promising. It should be started at 7.5 mg and increased to 15 mg daily. If clients are taking a generic folic acid supplement instead, it is a good idea for them to supplement it with vitamin B12 since folic acid masks symptoms of B12 deficiency. Deplin, on the other hand, does not have this problem. Clients with a BMI over 30 are also more likely to respond to Deplin, as are clients who have a history of eating disorders, kidney disease, alcohol use disorder, smoking, or are taking oral contraceptives (Shelton et al., 2015). Although Deplin requires a prescription, an over-the-counter form of l-methylfolate is now available.

Although stimulants and Provigil® (modafinil), a wakefulness-promoting agent, were previously recommended to augment antidepressants, recent studies have shown they are ineffective. Similarly, testosterone is not effective for augmenting antidepressants, though it does effectively treat low testosterone, which can present with symptoms that mimic depression. Finally, Lamictal® (lamotrigine), which is a mood stabilizer often used to treat bipolar disorders, is not effective for the treatment of depression.

Treatment-Resistant Depression

Treatment-resistant depression kills people, so keep asking about suicidality. Remember, you cannot tell if your client is suicidal simply by how they look. Fortunately, there are new options. In addition to prescription neurotransmitter-focused antidepressants, ketamine is a promising agent that improves depression immediately. It is a type of anesthetic medication that was initially developed for use in short medical procedures several decades ago. Ketamine is thought to treat depression immediately by promoting brain plasticity, although this is a theory, not a fact. Because of its dissociative qualities, ketamine is known colloquially as Special K and is abused for its hallucinogen properties. It is not entirely clear if this agent works on glutamate or opiate receptor sites. However, this and likely other agents being developed open a completely new mechanism (and hope) for clients with treatment-resistant depression.

Ask Your Client

For treatment-resistant depression, take time to review your client's daily routine regarding the critical five: nutrition, sleep, social connection, mindfulness practice, and exercise. There are manualized tools, such as WILD 5 Wellness®, that can help your client break down these important skills and habits into doable chunks with impressive outcome data (Cook et al., 2012).

In addition, take time to review for possible missed diagnoses. Is there an unaddressed anxiety or substance use disorder? Asking about and addressing these issues can help treatment for depression be more effective. Also make sure to keep an eye out for your client's exhaustion level by asking questions like, "Where are you at in terms of 'getting to the end of your rope?" Exhaustion is very connected to suicidality.

Finally, review whether a change in therapy approach may be more helpful. For example, for clients struggling with sleep, it may be helpful to use cognitive-behavioral therapy for insomnia (CBT-I) to augment and improve treatment for depression. Prolonged insomnia, agitation, and severe anxiety are the "lethal trio" for suicidal behaviors. What other non-medication options are there to consider, such as electroconvulsive therapy and trans-cranial magnetic stimulation? Communicating with your client's prescriber is critical in order to actively change the treatment plan.

When and How to Stop Antidepressants

On the other end of the treatment experience, when should your client stop their medication? Deprescribing is somewhat of a lost art, and your client may be left to decide on their own. The general principles are to **(1)** give the brain adequate time to function in a "non-depressed" mode (nine months to one year) before considering tapering an effective treatment, and **(2)** decrease the antidepressant very slowly while assuring daily wellness. If possible, the deprescribing process should also occur during a time in your client's life that presents with minimal distress and challenges. During this time, continuing with psychotherapy is very helpful, and maintaining good sleep is essential. Some clients also find it helpful to start one of the complementary agents described in Chapter 6.

If your client has had more than two depressive episodes in the past five years or more than three episodes in their lifetime (especially with suicidal behaviors, psychosis, or hospitalization), have a conversation in which you weigh the costs and benefits of discontinuing versus staying on medication. Once your client begins the process of tapering down their medication, you can either give them a blank PHQ-9 to monitor for early symptoms of depression or incorporate monitoring for new depressive symptoms during their therapy visits.

Antidepressants can cause substantial discomfort when rapidly discontinued, so warn your client against suddenly stopping the medication. The common symptoms of this possible antidepressant discontinuation syndrome are **F**lu-like symptoms, **I**nsomnia, **N**ausea, **I**mbalance, **S**ensory disturbances, and **H**yperarousal **(FINISH)**. Paxil (paroxetine), Effexor (venlafaxine), and Cymbalta (duloxetine) are particularly likely to cause this syndrome, but it has been documented in some clients for virtually all antidepressants. Prozac (fluoxetine), Wellbutrin (bupropion), and Remeron (mirtazapine) are less likely to trigger it.

Take care to explain to clients that this syndrome is not a reflection of being addicted to their antidepressant medication. It is the body's response to sudden drops in blood levels of the neurotransmitters. The "treatment" is to take the medication and taper off more slowly. Some clients will need to taper as slowly as 25 percent of the medication per month (Muzina, 2010). Most who have symptoms will find that they resolve in a week or two. Low-dose Prozac has been successfully used to prevent this syndrome while tapering down other antidepressants, as Prozac stays in the body longer and gradually dissipates.

Vulnerable Populations

Pregnant and Postpartum Women

Pregnancy is a high-risk time for developing or worsening an existing mood disorder. Even if a client has been stable on antidepressants and in complete remission, they have a 30 percent chance of getting depressed during pregnancy, even if they stay on their medication. If they decide to stop their antidepressant, then that risk more than doubles (Cohen et al., 2006). Deciding whether or not to discontinue antidepressant use during pregnancy is a difficult decision, and unfortunately there is not a "no risk" option. Maternal anxiety and depression negatively affect the health of a developing baby and can continue to affect cognitive and motor development into early childhood.

The treatment of choice for mild to moderate depression is psychotherapy. For clients with severe depression who require medication, antidepressants—with the exception of Paxil (paroxetine)—are considered relatively safe in pregnancy. The SSRIs and tricyclics have the most data for safety. In general, it is much better to increase the dose of an antidepressant if needed rather than to abandon it and try a second antidepressant. Pregnancy is one time when complementary agents (such as St. John's wort) are not recommended because their purity is not regulated by the FDA. Although antidepressants are associated with some risks during pregnancy, such as a slight increase in low birth weight and pre-term delivery, these events occur at about the same rate as babies born to mothers with untreated depression during pregnancy. There is no evidence of any long-term adversity from antidepressants other than Paxil, and there is clear evidence that antidepressants do not cause autism or ADHD (Sujan et al., 2017).

In addition to the prenatal period, the postnatal period is also a specific time of concern when it comes to mood disorders, as postpartum depression (PPD) affects 10 to 20 percent of new mothers. For those who have a baby in the neonatal intensive care unit, the rate skyrockets to 70 percent. The onset can occur during pregnancy and up to one month postpartum. And, yes, fathers can develop PPD too. In contrast to some other forms of depression, PPD often has a significant anxiety component, and the client's mood often presents as more labile than consistently sad.

Ask Your Client

Don't forget to ask about suicide. Suicide is a significant source of morbidity in postpartum women.

In women, PPD is believed to be caused or triggered by the dramatic hormonal changes involving estrogen and progesterone that occur postpartum. Therefore, the treatment of choice for PPD is a hormonal medication, Zulresso® (brexanolone), which is administered by a continuous IV over a 60-hour-period in a health care setting. Its administration is supervised according to protocols set up by the Risk Evaluation Management System, as mandated by the FDA. The concern is sudden sedation and loss of consciousness. Zulresso has been shown to improve depressive symptoms by the end of the two-and-a-half-day infusion, with these results continuing at a 30-day evaluation (Morrison et al., 2019).

In addition, sleep is essential to treatment of PPD (Stewart & Vigod, 2016). Work with your client to ensure she gets "more than enough" sleep. Doing so usually involves bringing in significant family members, friends, and other supports to make

Case Example

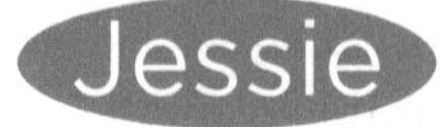

Jessie

Jessie was 14 years old when she was first prescribed Zoloft (sertraline) for severe depression. She was started at 50 mg daily, which is the full adult starting dose, and two days later she reported feeling better but "antsy." One week later, she couldn't sit still and felt like she "wanted to rip someone's head off." When a friend's mom angered her—in Jessie's words, "pissed me off"—Jessie and her friend impulsively overdosed on bottles of Advil® (ibuprofen) and Tylenol® (acetaminophen). Both girls survived without long-lasting adverse effects after emergency room treatment.

Following the incident, Jessie was switched to 5 mg of Celexa (citalopram), which is 25 percent of the adult dose. She was able to tolerate the medication without akathisia, so it was gradually increased to 20 mg daily. Her therapist was key in working with Jessie and her mom on increasing her sleep, assessing for akathisia, and encouraging her to continue her medication after it was working and she thought she no longer needed it.

sure she gets uninterrupted, quality sleep. Breastfeeding may need to be re-discussed with involvement of her pediatrician or nurse practitioner. No medication will treat PPD without good sleep.

Postpartum psychosis is another type of mental illness that can occur during the postpartum period, although it is much rarer. It occurs in about 1 out of every 1,000 women after birth but is considered a psychiatric emergency. If your client is exhibiting delusions following childbirth, especially around needing to protect the baby from harm, I recommend calling 911 for further evaluation in an emergency setting. Do not send your client home to pack a bag or for any other reason. This is the psychiatric equivalent of someone in cardiac arrest. Your client needs immediate intervention to prevent a potentially tragic outcome, such as suicide and infant injury or death.

Youth

Depression looks different in children, adolescents, and even young adults, as the brain does not fully develop until 25 years of age. Sad mood may or may not be present, and irritability is much more common. Therefore, the challenge in distinguishing depression from the initial onset of bipolar disorders involves ensuring an accurate differential diagnosis: grandiosity and increased goal-directed activity are symptoms highly indicative of bipolar disorders, whereas irritability is more likely associated with major depressive disorder and anxiety.

Although there are many causes of depression in youth, recent studies have linked depression and suicide with increased media and digital "screen time" and decreased sleep (Lin et al., 2016; Twenge et al., 2019). Therefore, the treatment of choice for adolescents with mild to moderate depression involves ensuring adequate sleep, proper nutrition, daily exercise, and decreased screen time (Radovic & Moreno, 2019). Psychotherapy is also effective, with CBT and interpersonal therapy exhibiting the best evidence. Medication alone is rarely the treatment of choice for youth. However, for moderate to severe depression, or when therapy and lifestyle changes have failed, SSRI antidepressants are the preferred choice of medication. Although SNRIs are also being prescribed to individuals under 25 years of age, there is less data supporting these agents. Tricyclics do not work for youth.

SSRIs need to be started at very low doses (10 to 25 percent of the usual adult starting dose) to prevent akathisia, to which the adolescent brain is highly sensitive. The agitation and irritability of akathisia combined with the hopelessness of teen depression can trigger impulsive suicidal behaviors, which explains why the biggest cause of the SSRI-related suicidality in youth is akathisia. Starting at a very low dose with SSRIs causes less akathisia and results in less impulsive suicidal behavior.

Older Adults

Depression looks different in older adults, as only 50 percent of this population exhibit sadness as a symptom of depression. Therefore, typical questionnaires or tools that measure sadness will fail to detect depression among many older clients.

Instead, the hallmark symptom of depression in older adults is cognitive change. For example, your client may become convinced someone is stealing their mail. These cognitive symptoms can be persistent and appear like dementia, which is why it is often termed "pseudodementia." Think depression first if you have a client with a history of depressive episodes who begins to exhibit cognitive changes.

Somatic complaints are also common among older adults. They may see their primary care provider more frequently with complaints of gastrointestinal upset, pain, and other concerns. While at their primary care provider, be sure your client is evaluated for a urinary tract infection, which can look like depression and even psychosis. If you are concerned an underlying infection may be contributing to your client's symptoms, you can send an electronic or faxed communication to their primary care provider describing the change you see in your client's presentation, and ask if there are any infections or other medical conditions that might be contributing. Be sure to include plenty of room on the page for a response if you fax your question.

SSRIs are also the first-line treatment for older adults with depression because these medications only affect serotonin. Medications that target norepinephrine can affect the heart rhythm and this is something to avoid in older adults, so medications such as SNRIs are generally not recommended (American Geriatrics Society Beers Criteria® Update Expert Panel, 2019). Tricyclic antidepressants are also problematic because their heavy anticholinergic burden can exacerbate cognitive impairment in older adults.

In contrast to youth, older adults rarely experience akathisia with SSRIs. In addition, they tend to tolerate sexual dysfunction better than younger clients. However, because of liver, kidney, and overall metabolic changes that occur with aging, the initial dose is still low and then slowly titrated as needed. "Start low, go slow" is the slogan of safe prescribing for older adults.

Because cognitive impairment is a common symptom of depression in older adults, Aricept® (donepezil) is the medication of choice if the SSRI needs augmentation. In this case, the Aricept is not treating dementia; it is treating depression. In fact, it is a myth that clients with dementia are likely to develop depression because of their condition. The reality is that it works the other way around. Recurrent depressive episodes increase the risk of developing cognitive impairment and dementia (James et al., 2018). Yet another important reason to treat depressive episodes to full remission.

Older adults with depression have poorer treatment outcomes, but it is possible to double the effectiveness of treatment by combining incremental, regular adjustments in medication dosage with problem-solving treatment (Unützer et al., 2002). Drawing on the principles of behavioral activation, one form of problem-solving treatment—known as Problem-Solving Treatment in Primary Care (PST-PC)—encourages older adults to come up with solutions to the life problems that are contributing to their depression by eliminating the source of the frustration or obsession. For example, the older client convinced someone is stealing their mail may find that changing their mailbox is helpful. By getting active and implementing a plan, clients increase their sense of self-efficacy in their ability to solve everyday problems.

Co-occurring Substance Use Disorders

Clients who have a substance use disorder in addition to depression tend to respond better to agents that target norepinephrine, such as the SNRIs, tricyclics, and Wellbutrin (bupropion). Having said that, if your client has done well on a particular antidepressant in the past, it is highly likely to work again—even if that medication only focuses on serotonin. Let the prescribing provider know about that! Your client may have forgotten to mention it in the anxiety and rush of the prescriber appointment.

Insomnia tends to be a big issue for clients with co-occurring depression and substance use, so I find many do well on Remeron (mirtazapine) given its sedating effect. They appreciate getting better sleep, do not experience akathisia, and often respond well to its antidepressant effect. Remember, the lowest dose is the most sedating. Remeron is also not lethal on overdose, nor is it dangerous combined with substances of abuse.

Wellbutrin is not recommended for clients who have alcohol use disorders, as there is an increased risk of seizures when they stop drinking. I also avoid using tricyclics with clients who are actively abusing substances; the danger of overdose is too high.

It is a myth that clients must be clean and sober before they will benefit from antidepressant medication. Oftentimes, the depressive symptoms seen among clients with a substance use disorder are indeed due to major depressive disorder, not only the demoralization seen with long-term addiction. Treating the underlying depression often helps clients experience a sense of hope that they can have a better life and supports recovery from substance use.

Conclusion

In summary, depression is common, disabling, and treatable. Talk with your client about medications when you know they are a good candidate. For example, if your client has a comorbid anxiety disorder, previous episodes of depression, a history of suicidal behaviors, or a family history of depression, you can confidently refer them to a prescribing provider to consider medication options that might work for them. Remember, your clients don't know that these agents really work, may be fearful of side effects, or believe that taking antidepressants means they're crazy. Stigma abounds. You play a critical role in motivating your client to consider medication, to hang in there while their provider finds the right medication, and to then stick with an effective medication regimen through the hassles of taking it. When it comes to depression, that can literally mean the difference between life and death.

Chapter 3

———

Treatment of Bipolar Disorders

Psychopharmacology for bipolar disorders has traditionally focused on treating existing (hypo)manic and depressive episodes as opposed to preventing new episodes. However, recurrent episodes of mania are associated with progressive deterioration in brain functioning over time (Abé et al., 2015). Because this cortical decline is correlated with the intensity, frequency, and length of episodes, long-term stability—that is, working to *prevent* new mood episodes and increase time without significant symptoms—is the new goal of treatment. This goal demands excellent psychotherapy and psychopharmacology, the use of empowering psychosocial strategies and support, and active collaboration between the client, therapist, psychiatric prescriber, and primary care provider.

Of course, the most critical participant is the client. Medications in bipolar disorders can be confusing, especially since optimal treatment for bipolar stability often requires multiple medications. Clients need to understand which agents are "anti-depression" and which are "anti-manic." Accordingly, this chapter provides you up-to-date information on medications and prioritized choices combined with practical strategies that improve the likelihood of treatment success, including:

- Which medications are first-line for which populations and why

- Which medications work best for (hypo)mania, depressive episodes, or both—and promote stability

- A useful metaphor that helps clients understand their medications and empowers them in their treatment

- Adverse effects to watch for

- How you can help your client identify problems and provide more useful information to their prescriber

- Strategies that increase the likelihood your clients will stay on medication that is working well, and what to do when they are becoming bored with stability

- Which agents are problematic to suddenly discontinue and how to help your client when they are thinking about stopping their medication

41

This chapter also presents you with information regarding the clinical use of anticonvulsant agents for other "vulnerable brain" states, such as traumatic brain injury, autism spectrum disorders, and agitation in dementia.

Helping Your Client Understand Their Medication

Psychiatric medication for bipolar disorders is complicated, but it's critical your client understands what each medication does in order to promote future stability and minimize further brain changes. To make it easier to understand, try using this metaphor: Some medications provide a floor, which keeps the client from falling into depressive episodes. Others provide a roof, which prevents them from blasting into (hypo)mania. Other medications provide both a floor and a roof. Still others treat symptoms, but don't prevent future episodes. That is, they get the client back into their living space, but don't keep them there.

This metaphor helps clients understand why when they become (hypo)manic—and go through the roof—it is helpful to take a "when you need it," or PRN, dose of a fast-acting atypical medication like Seroquel® (quetiapine), which has an excellent roof, as opposed to one that has an antidepressant or floor effect, like Lamictal (lamotrigine). When clients realize different medications have different purposes, they can come to a better understanding of why they take more than one pill. It also helps them make sense of changes recommended by their prescriber, which makes them more likely to follow through with those changes. Many of my clients return for their follow-up visits reporting success in using this metaphor. It seems to serve as a tool for increasing communication about the level of stability and the nature and intensity of mood episodes.

This metaphor is also helpful for clients who are eager to treat their depression but are reluctant to "lose" their mania or hypomania. Start with a floor; everyone agrees that's needed. From there, you can point out to your client that they also need a roof to keep stable and that they deserve to have that stability over time, not just today. Help your client see the connection between the cycles of (hypo)mania and depression. Ask them if they find intense depressive episodes follow times of mania or hypomania. This oscillating pattern is often the case. When they make that connection, many clients become motivated to aim for stability, even if it means losing (hypo)mania.

Treating Bipolar Disorders: The Agents

The classes of medications used to treat the bipolar disorders are lithium, anticonvulsants, and atypical antipsychotics—with antidepressants playing an adjunctive role. What makes a medication an excellent treatment for bipolar disorders is the degree to which it treats both acute (hypo)manic and depressive episodes, *and* prevents them from recurring, which is called maintenance. The ideal treatment for bipolar disorders addresses all four quadrants: (hypo)mania/ depression and treating/preventing. However, most medications do not.

Four Quadrants of Treatment

	Treats Current Episode	Prevents Future Episodes
(Hypo)Mania	Yes/No	Yes/No
Depression	Yes/No	Yes/No

The Canadian Network for Mood and Anxiety Treatments (CANMAT) international guidelines describe the effectiveness of different agents for the treatment and prevention of (hypo)mania and depression (Yatham et al., 2018). The tier-one level agents are summarized below. It's important to note that these lists are based on population data, meaning that the efficacy of these agents is determined by the percent of the population that gets well and stays well on that agent. Although these guidelines tell us which medications are most likely to work, your client may respond well on a second- or third-tier medication not on this list. Never argue with success.

CANMAT Tier-One Treatments for Adults with Bipolar Disorders

Brand Name	Generic Name	Treats Acute (Hypo) Mania	Treats Acute Depression	Prevents Future Episodes	Comments
Eskalith®, Lithobid ® (was)	Lithium	X	X	X	Can also be used for youth and older adults
Depakote®	Valproate	X	Some evidence	X	
Lamictal	Lamotrigine		X	X (Depression only)	
Seroquel	Quetiapine	X	X	X	
Latuda®	Lurasidone	X	X		
Vraylar®	Cariprazine	X	X	X	
Saphris®	Asenapine	X		X	
Invega®	Paliperidone	X			Dosages > 6 mg
Risperdal®	Risperidone	X			
Abilify®	Aripiprazole	X			
Tegretol®	Carbamazepine	X			

Lithium

Lithium, the first type of medication for bipolar disorders, is a natural salt and considered to be a first-line, or "gold standard," agent for the treatment of bipolar disorders. It both treats and prevents (hypo)mania and depressive episodes, and it significantly reduces rehospitalization rates compared to other medications

(Lähteenvuo et al., 2018; Post, 2018). Its effectiveness tends to continue for clients across decades, but it's underutilized. This underutilization is, in part, due to client fears of toxicity and the requirement for several blood draws a year. More significantly, though, lithium is underused because it is inexpensive and therefore not promoted by pharmaceutical companies (Bauer et al., 2016; Severus et al., 2014). Because of this minimal financial gain, you are also unlikely to see any media advertisements or new FDA indications for lithium, which are highly dependent on trials done by pharmaceutical companies.

In addition to being an excellent mood stabilizer, lithium is neuroprotective. Long-term use of lithium appears to protect the brain from structural changes in the amygdala and hippocampus associated with bipolar disorders (Machado-Vieira, 2009). No other medication protects against these progressive, structural changes. Lithium is also associated with lower rates of Alzheimer's disease, and it delays progression from mild cognitive impairment to dementia in clients with and without bipolar disorders (Forlenza et al., 2014; Morlet et al., 2018).

More than any other medication, lithium decreases suicidality and prevents future suicidality in clients with both depression and bipolar disorders (Lewitzka et al., 2015). If you have any client who exhibits suicidality, has a history of multiple suicidal episodes, or struggles with chronic suicidal ideation, they deserve to be considered for lithium treatment. Lithium decreases suicidality independent of its efficacy in treating the underlying depressive episode, although it does treat that too (see Augmentation section in Chapter 2).

However, some clients are not good candidates for lithium. These include individuals with renal (kidney) disease (or those who have only one kidney), those who are pregnant or want to get pregnant, those with cardiac conditions or psoriasis (it can aggravate these conditions), or those who are unable or unwilling to get regular blood draws.

Challenges with Lithium

Despite its efficacy, many clients are fearful of lithium because they have heard and worry about lithium toxicity. While the dose at which lithium is therapeutic versus toxic is very close—meaning it has a narrow therapeutic index—the good news is lithium toxicity is not difficult to detect. The symptoms of lithium toxicity are nausea, vomiting, and diarrhea. Lithium toxicity is not like hypertension, a condition that can kill you without symptoms, which is what clients fear. Explain this to your clients. You can decrease their fear and increase their motivation to seriously consider lithium as an option when it is suggested by their prescribing professional.

Case Example

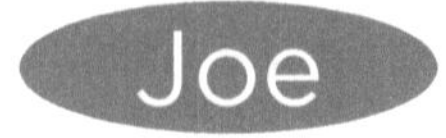

Joe, a 41-year-old man diagnosed with bipolar disorder, struggled with chronic suicidal thoughts, and his history of suicidal behavior had resulted in four psychiatric hospitalizations over the years. He had been on various medications for the treatment of bipolar disorders without success, including Depakote (valproate—caused weight gain), Risperdal (risperidone—didn't like the dystonia and weight gain), and antidepressants (didn't work).

He was now on Abilify (aripiprazole), which was controlling his mood swings, but he still struggled with suicidal thoughts every morning. He had not tried lithium and was worried it would make him sick. After some discussion, he agreed on a trial.

Two weeks later, he returned and reported he had a new problem: "I don't know what to do in the morning." What a most unusual visit "complaint"! He then elaborated that for the past week or so, when he would wake in the morning, the suicidal thoughts were just "gone." For years, he had spent the first several hours of every day talking himself into living instead of killing himself.

Suddenly, he had nothing to do. Such a wonderful problem. The success of lithium in treating his suicidality has been continuing for over two years.

Ask Your Client

- "What has been your experience with lithium?"

- "Did you know it's a natural salt? And did you know some natural hot springs contain lithium? Soaking there for a day or two does amazing things for your outlook on life!"

- "Have you ever been offered lithium, one of the very best treatments for bipolar disorders?"

- "It's okay if you are not interested. I just wanted you to know it is a 'best treatment' option."

- If they have concerns about toxicity, take them seriously. Then, explain how toxicity first presents itself as nausea, vomiting, and diarrhea. Let them know that recognizing these symptoms is what keeps them from getting toxic and that you can remind them which symptoms to watch out for if they forget.

As with any medication, lithium does have the potential for adverse effects. Some occur soon after starting lithium and are easily addressed; others occur over time and are only identified through blood draw results. Some of the adverse effects that can occur soon after starting lithium include nausea immediately after taking the medication, tremor, weight gain, cognitive dulling, and increased urination. More seriously, thyroid and renal (kidney) impairment can occur.

The nausea that some individuals experience after taking lithium is not due to stomach irritation; it reflects a mini-toxic episode. Since lithium is a natural salt, it is immediately absorbed into the bloodstream when taken on an empty stomach and can cause a sudden spike in the amount of lithium in the blood, similar to the toxicity if the dose is too high. This unwanted side effect can be prevented by taking lithium with food or by taking an extended- or sustained-release formulation of the medication. There is also a formulation that doesn't release until the medication is in the intestine, which is another way to prevent lithium levels from peaking too quickly.

In addition, a non-dangerous but annoying hand tremor can occur with lithium. For example, your client may notice hand shakiness that affects their handwriting or causes them to spill their morning coffee. Ask your clients if they experience this side effect and, if so, whether it is problematic. Clients will likely discontinue the medication unless this issue is addressed. Fortunately, the tremor can be decreased or eliminated with propranolol, which is a blood pressure medication that decreases jitteriness without affecting brain function. Encourage clients to contact their prescribing provider if the tremors become bothersome and not to stop their lithium. It is also worth noting that benzodiazepines, such as Klonopin® (clonazepam), are not the first-line treatment for this tremor.

> ## *Alert Your Client*
>
> Propranolol is used for both performance anxiety (stage fright) and for anxiety related to sudden exposure to trauma. It decreases jitteriness, stomach butterflies, and sweaty palms, and it slows heart rate, all without affecting brain function. Benzodiazepines, on the other hand, decrease cognitive anxiety while negatively affecting motor functioning, such as the ability to drive a motor vehicle. Benzodiazepines also block the brain's ability to process trauma during sleep, which increases the risk of post-traumatic stress disorder (PTSD).

Lithium can also cause some weight gain, although the actual amount varies significantly from person to person and is less than many of the other agents used for treating bipolar disorders. Have a conversation with your client about fears of weight gain with lithium. For clients who have reason to worry, it can be helpful to have them track their actual weight gain. Doing so allows them to predict their anticipated weight gain and then test that prediction by measuring the actual impact. When weight gain occurs, and some gain is common, it occurs early in treatment and then tends to level out. It is uncommon for it to continue to increase. In my experience, I have found that clients who have had many years of instability find the stability of life on lithium so desirable that they decide to manage their weight in other ways and continue the medication.

> ## *Alert Your Client*
>
> Clients should never suddenly discontinue lithium unless directed by their prescriber. If anything is problematic, encourage your clients to talk with their prescriber about an alternative medication and how to taper off the lithium. Abruptly stopping lithium greatly increases the risk of (hypo)mania, depression, and suicidal thoughts.

Cognitive dulling, or a sensation of not being as sharp as usual, is uncommon with lithium but does occur. This adverse effect waxes and wanes over time and can be addressed with supplemental thyroid hormone. Frequent urination can also occur. Encourage your client to talk with their prescriber if they experience this symptom. Often, it is a benign problem, but it can be more serious if it is interrupting your client's sleep.

Finally, lithium can have serious adverse effects on thyroid and renal (kidney) functioning, which is why clients must be monitored by lab tests that require regular blood draws. It is critical to monitor thyroid and renal functioning when lithium is started, a month or so later, and then two to three times a year. Although many clients are afraid that lithium requires blood draws "all the time," that perception is inaccurate. However, periodic blood draws are critical for safety.

Thyroid impairment presents as low energy, depressed mood, and other physical changes (e.g., dry skin, hair loss, hoarse voice, brittle nails) and is recognized by a blood test and physical exam evaluating the size of the thyroid gland. The current recommendation in the case of impaired thyroid functioning is to treat it with thyroid supplementation and continue treatment with lithium since bipolar disorders are a life-threatening illness with few options.

Renal (kidney) impairment is a different story. When lithium affects the kidneys, the impairment worsens over time, but your client will not exhibit symptoms until after significant damage has occurred. The risk of kidney damage is the primary reason clients must absolutely get regular blood draws. Approximately two percent of people on lithium will develop kidney failure if they continue to take lithium, so if your client experiences any adverse impacts on their kidneys, they need to stop taking lithium. Lithium is least impactful on kidney functioning when the entire dose is taken once daily.

Ask Your Client

"How long has it been since you've had your blood drawn?" If it has been over six months, refer them to their prescriber. Save your client time and hassle by contacting the prescribing provider and asking, "Do you want me to tell our client to go to the lab first, or wait for an appointment to see you?" Doing so can save your client significant time and extra health care visits.

Determining the "Right" Dose

Effectiveness and the "right" dose are determined by a combination of clinical improvement and your client's blood level. It is not determined by the number of pills they take. It is critical to combine these two factors to truly assess improvement because the goal of treatment is not for your client to feel better today; it is for them to continue feeling better today, next week, next month, and so on. You get the idea. When you see your client on a particular day, it only gives you a snapshot in time of how they are doing, which is important but not sufficient to ensure stability. Two weeks from your visit, your client may become manic or depressed if their blood level is inadequate. Remember, even clients with bipolar disorder who are unmedicated are euthymic about 50 percent of the time. But the other 50 percent devastates their lives.

The greatest difficulty in determining the right dose has to do with the time of day your client gets their blood drawn. The most effective and safest dose of lithium is determined by the results from blood drawn 12 hours after taking lithium. Not 9 hours, not 15 hours—it must be 12 hours (+/– *only 1 hour*) in order for the results to be accurate enough to optimize therapy with lithium. Getting lithium levels drawn at the wrong time is a common cause of error in decision making about the right dose. When the blood is drawn too soon after taking lithium, it creates a falsely elevated level. When it is drawn too long after, the opposite effect occurs. Either way, it may cause the prescriber to change the dose and destabilize or cause toxicity in your client.

Help your clients figure out specifics to maximize the effectiveness (and accuracy) of their blood draws. Ask your client what times they usually take their lithium, and plan how they can get to the lab at 12 hours post-dose. If they take their lithium in the morning, exactly how do they intend to get their blood drawn at 9 p.m.? Clients who take lithium in the morning will need to switch to taking it during the evening or at bedtime for a few days until the blood draw is complete. They can then resume taking it every morning if they'd like. One final tip: If your client takes lithium twice a day, then the blood draw should still occur 12 hours after a dose. Remind your client to not take their morning dose until after they get their blood drawn. If they forget and take their pill, then they should skip the blood draw and do it another day.

Alert Your Client

1. It is critical that your clients periodically get their blood drawn to ensure that their lithium levels are safe. Two to three times a year is the usual frequency, with slightly more blood draws required when there are dosing changes.

2. It is important to watch for the "trio of toxicity": nausea, vomiting, and diarrhea. Any one of these symptoms without obvious cause (e.g., your client's child or coworkers are sick with the flu, or the whole family got food poisoning after eating out) requires a call to the prescribing provider pronto.

3. Educate your client on the importance of asking their prescriber, "If I feel any of the toxic trio symptoms, what do you want me to do until I can get a hold of you?" You want your clients to know what to do immediately in the event that these symptoms occur. Make a note of the agreed-upon plan so you can remind them of it if needed.

Therapeutic benefit requires blood levels between 0.6 to 1.2 mEq/l, though older adults tend to require levels slightly lower than that (0.4 to 0.6 mEq/l). Generally, the most optimal level is the lowest within that range, which provides mood stability without (hypo)mania or depression over time. (Hypo)mania often responds to doses in this lower therapeutic range, but clients with depression often need 0.8 mEq/l or higher (Yatham et al., 2018). The dose of lithium needed to get to a therapeutic level varies by individual. A common lithium dose is between 600 to 1500 mg daily, but some clients need only 300 to 450 mg daily, while others need 2100 mg.

Remember, the critical number is the blood level, not how much medication your client is taking, in combination with clinical improvement. For example, I will sometimes increase lithium even though the level is "therapeutic" at 0.7 mEq/l because the client still feels irritable and their mood is fluctuating—all indicators that they are unstable. After I increase the dose and their blood level rises to 0.9 mEq/l, they become less depressed, less irritable, and more stable. For this client, a higher dose is more therapeutic. On the other hand, if I have a client who reports that they feel better, are no longer experiencing mood swings, and are able to function well in life at a level of 0.7 mEq/l, then I do not increase the dose. Clinical picture and blood level provide the most effective determination of the dose needed for optimal stability.

In addition, your client's lithium level can change over time, even when nothing else has changed. The level is impacted by the amount of nicotine or caffeine, dehydration, and significant increases or decreases in the use of ibuprofen and other nonsteroidal anti-inflammatory drugs. (Taking an ibuprofen once in a while does not count.) Therefore, if you have a client with bipolar disorder who is exhibiting worsening depressive symptoms, communicate your observations with their prescriber. It is highly likely they will want an updated lithium level on your client. To reduce the hassle for your client, ask the prescriber whether they want you to send the client to the lab to get their lithium level drawn first, or wait to schedule a follow-up visit. Remind your client when and how to get their blood drawn. Do not tolerate ongoing depressive symptoms being "as good as it gets."

Anticonvulsants

The second category of medications for the treatment of bipolar disorders are the anticonvulsants. However, not all anticonvulsants treat bipolar disorders, so do not assume your client is being treated for bipolar disorder simply because they are on Keppra® (levetiraceam) for seizures. Only Depakote (valproate, valproic acid, or divalproex sodium), Lamictal (lamotrigine), Tegretol (carbamazepine), and Trileptal® (oxcarbazepine) are useful in the treatment of bipolar disorders.

Ask Your Client

All anticonvulsants have a black box warning indicating that they can increase the risk of suicidality. This increased risk is independent of mood, so regularly ask any clients taking an anticonvulsant about suicidality.

Depakote

Depakote is rarely referred to by its generic names (valproate, valproic acid, or divalproex sodium) even when the generic formulation is being used. It is considered an effective top-tier agent for the treatment and prevention of both hypomania and mania (Yatham et al., 2018), though it can also be helpful in treating depressive episodes. However, depression often requires higher doses than (hypo)mania.

Depakote can be used concurrently with lithium or atypical antipsychotics and is often used in combination with these agents to promote full mood stabilization. However, it does have drug interactions with Tegretol and Lamictal that require special care and attention. When either of these combinations are used, it becomes paramount to watch for a rash indicative of Stevens-Johnson syndrome (see section on Lamictal) and to get regular blood draws because taking one medication affects the blood level of the other in complex ways.

Some older studies suggest that Depakote works best with clients who have rapid cycling bipolar disorder or a concurrent substance use disorder (Calabrese et al., 2001), although this information is less influential in determining prescription guidelines. Prescribers now determine which agent to prescribe based on studies of efficacy, what adverse effects they need to avoid, what other symptoms can be treated at the same time, and what other factors might impact treatment (e.g., insurance coverage and family or personal history of medication response). A comprehensive Cochrane Review found that Depakote works best to prevent future episodes of (hypo)mania and depression when combined with lithium (Cipriani et al., 2013).

Similar to lithium, Depakote dosing is dependent on blood level. The timing of the blood draw is not quite as particular as is the case with lithium, though, as the draw can occur anywhere from 10 to 12 hours after the last dose. Generally, (hypo)mania responds to blood levels above 50 µg/mL, while depressive symptoms (when they do respond) require a level above 80 µg/mL.

Other Uses of Anticonvulsants

Depakote (valproate) and Tegretol (carbamazepine) can be very useful in treating the sudden rage associated with intermittent explosive disorder, as well as the irritability and agitation seen in autism spectrum disorders, dementia, sequelae from traumatic brain injury, and other disruptive behavioral states. It is preferred over the use of antipsychotics for behavior management when there is no evidence of psychosis. Usually low doses, such as 250 mg of Depakote twice daily, are effective. Doses can be even lower for older adults or children with conditions requiring behavioral management. For example, Depakote comes in 125 mg "sprinkles" that can be put in food.

Depakote is more sedating than lithium and has a slight anti-anxiety effect. It can be taken once daily or multiple times a day to manage this effect. Clients with anxiety or benzodiazepine use disorders tend to like taking it multiple times daily; clients with insomnia generally prefer taking it at bedtime.

In addition to sedation, other common adverse effects include dizziness, weight gain, and (less commonly) nausea, vomiting, abdominal pain, and difficulty with coordination. Any client on Depakote with significant abdominal pain should be referred to their prescriber, as this can be an indication of pancreatitis, a life-threatening condition usually requiring hospitalization. For this reason, clients with a history of pancreatitis should never take Depakote.

Depakote is also stressful on the liver, so clients with cirrhosis or severe hepatic disease need particularly close monitoring when prescribed this agent. It can also cause changes in blood cell production involving reduced platelet count, which can interfere with clients' ability to fight infections. Both of these serious adverse effects are monitored with regular blood draws, generally twice yearly.

Infrequently, but at any point in time, Depakote can increase the amount of ammonia in the blood and brain. Ammonia neurotoxicity causes fatigue, sedation, and confusion. It will appear as if your client is heavily sedated on drugs, even falling asleep, and cognitively confused. You should communicate these observations to the prescriber right away. The prescriber may email or fax directions immediately back to you, or call the client directly. If you cannot connect with the prescriber, the client should contact their prescriber's after hours or urgent care resources for directions.

Depakote also causes problems specific to women. For example, ten percent of women experience polycystic ovary syndrome within the first year of taking Depakote, which is a condition associated with hormonal changes, weight gain, and a six-fold increased risk of developing diabetes mellitus II. Depakote is also highly teratogenic and contains a black box warning because of its potential risk for birth defects, including significant impairments in behavioral and cognitive functioning (Cohen et al., 2019; Velez-Ruiz & Meador, 2015). Therefore, it should be only taken by women of childbearing capacity when it is essential for the treatment of the bipolar disorder—that is, when all other agents have failed or are contraindicated. When that is the case, your client must be on effective birth control. You are likely to see women of childbearing capacity who are still being prescribed Depakote who may not be aware of this risk. Let them know. They should talk with their prescriber and not simply stop taking Depakote. The website womensmentalhealth.org is another excellent site for their reference.

Alert Your Client

Depakote (valproate) comes in regular, delayed-release, and extended-release formulations. The regular formulation is rarely used. When switching from the more commonly prescribed delayed-release to extended-release tablets, your client will have a drop of 20 to 25 percent medication when taking the same dose. Therefore, in order to stay stable and keep the same blood level, the dose needs to be increased by approximately 25 percent when switching to extended-release tablets. Alert your client to this information if they have their Depakote changed.

Lamictal

Lamictal is a medication with a strong antidepressant effect (e.g., a good floor) and is an excellent agent for clients who have experienced significant, protracted depressive episodes as part of their bipolar disorder. It is especially useful for clients with bipolar II disorder, who experience oscillating periods of depression and hypomania (as opposed to mania). Clients with bipolar disorder who experience significant anxiety also do well on Lamictal.

However, Lamictal does not provide significant protection from mania, so it is not considered a medication with a good roof. Clients with a history of mania, and those with significant episodes of hypomania, will likely need Lamictal combined with another medication that targets (hypo)manic symptoms. I rely solely on Lamictal only when a client has a history of a few hypomanic episodes—with perhaps years between them—and they are very clear about what the initial symptoms of getting hypomanic involve. I give them a prescription for an atypical agent to keep on hand and instruct them to take it at the first sign of hypomania and call me.

There are advantages to Lamictal. It causes little to no weight gain, and clients do not need to get regular blood draws. It also isn't overly sedating or activating. However, Lamictal requires a lengthy titration to decrease the likelihood of developing Stevens-Johnson syndrome, which is a very serious, potentially life-threatening skin reaction that can be triggered by Lamictal (and other medications as well). This syndrome begins with a rash, which is obvious in nature and does not just resemble a few pimples. Gradually increasing the dose is very important, as it decreases the likelihood your client will have this problem.

The rash can occur anytime, although the highest incidence is during the titration phase, as well as if the dose gets increased later during treatment. If your client has a rash, they need to talk with their provider right away. The rash is not considered a medical emergency, so they shouldn't go to urgent care, but they need to see their provider immediately. When your client contacts their prescriber, they are likely to be told to discontinue the medication, but the provider may ask to see the client to evaluate the rash rather than immediately stopping the medication. By asking your client if they have a rash, you increase the safety of prescribing Lamictal.

Because of its prolonged titration period, Lamictal is less useful for depressive symptoms that require a more rapid treatment response. Even clients with a long history of depressive episodes can become discouraged by the slow titration process. With a few exceptions, the starting dose is 25 mg daily for two weeks, followed by 50 mg for another two weeks, and eventually 100 mg. Some clients respond at 100 mg, but they often need 200 mg, which requires further titration. You can see how this process can be frustrating for a client in the midst of a depressive episode. Sometimes, clients don't want to give the medication a trial because of the lengthy dosing process.

If your client's prescriber suggests they try Lamictal but they are discouraged by it "taking two months to work," you can help motivate your client. In this situation, ask your client, "Would you say that depression has been a recent problem in your life, or has it been a problem for a long time?" When they endorse it as a long-term issue, you can follow up with, "So maybe it's time to consider something that will prevent depression in the future *and* get rid of it now. You can think of Lamictal as a kind of investment: It takes time to build, but when you get there, it's likely to keep working a long time." This conversation can also assist clients during the titration period by encouraging them not to give up or attempt to increase their dose faster than prescribed.

Lamictal works well in combination with other agents, such as lithium or atypical antipsychotics. However, it must be added carefully to Depakote due to the increased potential for Stevens-Johnson syndrome, or elevated blood levels of both agents due to drug interactions between the two. Lamictal may also decrease the effectiveness of oral birth control pills, the patch, and the vaginal ring. These forms of birth control also decrease the amount of lamotrigine available in the body, so a client who is started on oral contraceptives may become more depressed and pregnant as well. Your client either needs to be on a higher dose of Lamictal to counter this interaction or be on a different combination of medications altogether. Lamictal does not impair the emergency contraceptive pill.

Lamictal can be taken once daily at any time your client prefers. Some people find it slightly energizing; others find it mildly sedating. When your client has had a good response to Lamictal and then months later has worsened mood, contact their prescriber. Frequently, a small increase in dose can help the Lamictal kick in again. Do not accept worsening or ongoing depressive symptoms as inevitable. Communicate your observation of worsened mood, including suicidality or lack thereof, and whether your client has been regularly taking their medication(s). Including your client's pharmacy and lab preference is always a good idea. You can also ask whether your client should make an appointment, and if the prescriber wants to make any changes while your client is waiting for the appointment.

Alert Your Client

If your client misses more than a few days of Lamictal (lamotrigine), they should contact their prescriber or pharmacy. They will likely need to start the titration process all over again, beginning at 25 mg. Directly resuming their full therapeutic dose increases the risk of Stevens-Johnson syndrome.

Tegretol

Tegretol is considered a second- or third-tier agent, but it works well for some clients. If your client is euthymic and stable on this medication, do not argue with success. For clients who respond, it is more effective as a "roof" in treating and protecting against (hypo)mania than it is for treating or preventing depression. Tegretol does not cause any problems with weight gain, and it can be used by women of childbearing capacity since it does not pose the risk of birth defects seen with Depakote. It does, however, require blood draws to screen for impact on liver functioning and blood cell production. As with lithium and Depakote, the effective dose of Tegretol is determined by efficacy and blood level, not by dose of the medication.

Trileptal

Trileptal is a derivative of the active ingredient in Tegretol, which is carbamazepine. Because it has less data supporting its effectiveness for both (hypo)mania and depression, it is considered a third- or fourth-tier agent. However, if your client responds well on Trileptal and maintains stability without any adverse effects, then it may be a great option for them. Trileptal also has less adverse effects on blood cell production, so it does not require the blood draws of Tegretol.

Atypical Antipsychotics

Atypical antipsychotics are the third class of medications used to treat bipolar disorders. Most atypical agents effectively treat and prevent mania, and some also treat and prevent depression, regardless if there is any psychosis. Clients do not need to be psychotic to benefit from these medications, which is why these antipsychotics are often referred to as atypical "agents"; they do more than treat psychosis.

All atypical agents require blood draws to monitor their impact on blood glucose and lipid levels several times a year. The adverse effects, including the amount of weight gain and level of sedation, vary greatly between the atypical agents. However, one distinct advantage of this class of medications as a whole is that they work quickly and can be added to other medications on a PRN basis to rapidly decrease the onset of mania, and even to stem early depressive symptoms. These agents work very well in combination with lithium, Depakote, Tegretol, and Lamictal. Frequently, your clients will need more than one medication to get optimal treatment.

Timing is everything when improving stability. Clients need to have their medication available at any time—not when the clinic opens or when they have an appointment with their provider. They need to be able to respond quickly when they experience early symptoms of deterioration, as doing so significantly increases stability and decreases the suffering, dysfunction, and hospitalizations associated with (hypo)manic episodes. Clients experience more control over and efficacy in managing their illness, which motivates them to stay on medication.

Ask Your Client

Ask your client how they know when they are starting to get (hypo)manic. What is the very first thing they notice? Use their language for describing these changes (e.g., "What changes when you start to cycle up?"). Oftentimes, the first symptoms of instability involve changes in sleep and an increased motivation to "get things done"—both of which can feel good. Help your client connect these first symptoms to (hypo)mania and develop a safety plan. "What are the first two things you want to do when you notice this happening?" Hopefully, this list includes taking a PRN dose of an atypical agent. If not, encourage your client to ask their prescriber about this as a resource for "strengthening the roof" in particular.

Some atypical agents are also available in an injectable, long-acting formulation. Long-acting injectables are significantly more effective at keeping clients euthymic, stable, and out of the hospital (Lähteenvuo et al., 2018). In the past, these injections were only viewed as a treatment option for clients with poor insight and poor adherence to medication, but that is no longer the case. These medications are highly effective for any client, even more so than daily oral medication. Even the most dedicated clients forget their medication at times or can't remember if they took it last night or earlier tonight—so they skip it. Not to mention the hassle of running out of pills, needing to get to the pharmacy, and dealing with other life stressors that can interfere with taking a pill every day. It turns out many clients prefer and appreciate the convenience of just getting a shot once a month, so make sure your client is aware of this option for the treatment of bipolar disorders.

Additional information regarding specific types of atypical antipsychotics, including information on monthly injectables and their effectiveness for the phases of bipolar disorders, will be reviewed in Chapter 4.

Treating Depressive Episodes in Bipolar Disorders

Depressive symptoms in bipolar disorders are ubiquitous, disabling, and challenging to treat. In the past, the treatment of choice involved adding an antidepressant medication. However, antidepressants are usually less effective than other mood stabilizing agents and should generally be reserved for clients when other options have failed. Clients with a history of agitation or hypomania while on antidepressants should also not take these medications (Pacchiarotti et al., 2013).

The first strategy to treat depressive symptoms in bipolar disorders is to optimize the current mood stabilizing agent. For clients taking lithium, Depakote (valproate), or Tegretol (carbamazepine), that often means getting a current, 12-hour post-dose blood level. For clients prescribed atypical agents or Lamictal (lamotrigine), getting a blood level can also be helpful to identify rapid metabolizers and determine when

Ask Your Client

In order to assess your client's sleep, do a 24-hour sleep inventory, and count all time they spend with feet up (e.g., on the couch, sitting awake in bed) as sleep time. The circadian rhythm relies heavily on physical body position to determine sleep and wake cycles. Some questions to ask include:

- "What time do you go to bed? And what time do you actually fall asleep?"

- "When do you wake up?" (If they wake up in the night, ask how long they stay awake, as less than 15 minutes does not count as an awakening for the brain.)

- "When do you wake up next? And when do you get out of bed?"

- "Do you lie down or put your feet up in the daytime because you feel so exhausted?" (Adding the part about feeling "exhausted" encourages your client to include their time spent napping when they perhaps know that is frowned upon. While you are at it, assess for the use of stimulants in your 24-hour review.)

If clients need help improving their sleep, CBT-I is highly effective. Excellent resources on CBT-I are readily available. For clients, a good option is *Insomnia Solved: A Self-Directed Cognitive Behavioral Therapy for Insomnia (CBTI) Program* (Peters, 2018). For clinicians, a good resource is *Cognitive Behavioral Treatment of Insomnia: A Session by Session Guide* (Perlis, Jungquist, Smith, & Posner, 2008).

It is also important to differentiate sleep phase disorder (sleeping from 4 a.m. to noon after lying in bed for five hours trying to sleep) from insomnia. Youth naturally have a later sleep phase pattern, whereas older adults have an earlier sleep phase pattern. For some clients, insomnia may be connected to their attempts to override their natural sleep pattern.

In addition, I often use medication to assist clients with sleep. Atypical antipsychotics that have a sedating effect can be of use here, especially those that have an antidepressant effect. The short-term use of sleeping pills, such as Restoril® (temazepam) or Ambien® (zolpidem), is also effective provided there are no contraindications. Finally, melatonin is helpful (anywhere from 0.5 mg to 15 mg), but it needs to be taken several hours before bedtime, not at bedtime. The extended-release formulations help clients stay asleep, as well as fall asleep. Melatonin is the treatment of choice for youth and older adults.

the depressive symptoms are a result of irregular medication adherence. Frequently, adjusting the dose of the current medication based on the blood level results is enough to resolve the depressive episode and restore euthymia without having to add yet another medication. It generally takes a few weeks for the new dosage to "kick in."

In addition, the role of sleep is often overlooked. It is impossible to effectively treat depressive episodes or maintain stability when your client is not sleeping well. While I am waiting a few days for the blood level results, I focus on sleep. Again, get into the details.

If adjusting the dose of the current medication proves ineffective, other strategies include adding Lamictal or lithium, increasing the dose of an atypical agent, or adding or changing the atypical agent. Of the atypicals, four have FDA approval for treating depression in bipolar disorders: Seroquel (quetiapine), Vraylar (cariprasine), Latuda (lurasidone), and Zyprexa® (olanzapine) when it is combined with Prozac (fluoxetine). Lithium, Lamictal, Seroquel, Vraylar, and Latuda with lithium or Depakote are top-tier choices, whereas the combination of Zyprexa and Prozac is second-tier because of its propensity to cause serious weight gain (Yatham et al., 2018). For bipolar II disorder, Seroquel, lithium, and Lamictal are the top three agents. Wellbutrin (bupropion) in conjunction with lithium or Depakote—or, alternatively, Zoloft (sertraline) alone or with lithium or Depakote— are options when the top three have failed or have contraindications. A non-prescription alternative is N-acetylcysteine (NAC), which is an over-the-counter antioxidant with proven effectiveness in treating depressive symptoms in bipolar disorders. Additional information regarding NAC can be found in Chapter 6.

What about the use of antidepressants for clients with bipolar disorders who are currently depressed? Certainly, they are widely used and are helpful in certain circumstances. However, they can also be ineffective or even harmful and, in general, should not be used as the first option. According to the International Society for Bipolar Disorders, the following guidelines should be used when considering the use of antidepressants for the treatment of depressive episodes in bipolar disorders (Pacchiarotti et al., 2013):

1. Avoid all antidepressants if there are any "mixed" features in the midst of the depressive episode—such as agitation, racing thoughts, or irritability—or if the client has a history of mixed episodes.

2. Avoid antidepressants if the client is rapid cycling or has many episodes of mood swings.

3. Avoid antidepressants if they have ever triggered mania or hypomania.

4. Discontinue antidepressant medication if the client begins to exhibit mixed features.

5. Antidepressants may be prescribed for clients with bipolar II disorder if they have (1) had a sustained, positive response in the past to an antidepressant; (2) no mixed features; and (3) no history of agitation or hypomania on antidepressants. Antidepressants may be prescribed as monotherapy

(e.g., the only medication) if all these criteria are met and the client is regularly monitored.

6. Avoid all antidepressants for clients with bipolar I disorder who are not on a mood stabilizer, such as lithium, an atypical agent, or an anticonvulsant.

7. Discontinue the antidepressant after the mood has returned to euthymia (a state of feeling well) about two to three months after full remission, unless the client relapses into depression every time the antidepressant is stopped.

When a client is appropriate for an antidepressant (according to these guidelines), SSRIs are considered top-line choices, as these medications are less likely to cause agitation or (hypo)mania compared to SNRIs and tricyclics (Antosik-Wójcińska et al., 2015). However, some studies have found Paxil (paroxetine) ineffective. Another guideline recommends Zoloft (sertraline), Wellbutrin (bupropion), or Effexor (venlafaxine) as the best choices (Yatham et al., 2018). Studies also consistently list Prozac in combination with Zyprexa as effective. The specific medication that works best differs across individuals, so if your client has a history of doing well on a particular antidepressant without (hypo)mania or agitation, communicate that to the prescriber. That is *very* important information that sometimes gets missed either because the client forgets, or the prescriber doesn't ask in the pressure of a short medication visit.

With some exceptions, antidepressants can be stopped after your client is euthymic without triggering a relapse into depression. Although clients may be fearful about stopping the medication and credit it with having saved their life, clinical studies have found no differences in treatment outcomes between clients who stay on antidepressants versus those who taper off. In addition, there is some evidence that ongoing exposure to antidepressants roughens the stability of bipolar disorders. Educate your client about this information, and encourage them to discuss with their prescriber when (and if) they should taper off an antidepressant. Caution your client against suddenly stopping the medication or tapering off without consulting and coordinating with their prescriber. Sudden changes can trigger mood swings. The good news is there is no evidence that stopping antidepressants makes them less effective in the future.

Ultimately, when it comes to treating depression in bipolar disorders, if the medication your client is taking is not working, either the dose or the medication itself likely needs to be changed. What matters is what is tolerable and works for your client. Do not let your client settle for living in a partially depressed state. It can become the "new norm" and increases risk of eventual suicide.

Case Example

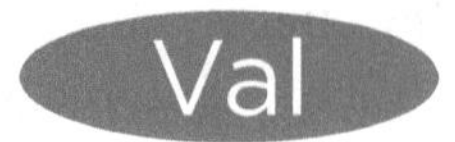

Val, who was 51 years old, suffered with bipolar II disorder with debilitating depressive episodes. She came to me on Zoloft (sertraline) and Seroquel (quetiapine), having been stable and euthymic for several years. After seeing her for about a year, we began to talk about tapering down her Zoloft. She was very anxious and believed she needed to stay on Zoloft indefinitely to prevent a relapse into depression.

I encouraged her to consider tapering off by first agreeing that the medication had worked. I asked her if she was currently depressed, to which she replied she was not. I then responded, "Then let's save it for when you need it. If you get depressed again, even a little bit, we'll immediately pull it back in." Val agreed to slowly decrease her dose.

Over the next four months, we slowly tapered her off. During this time, she continued on Seroquel and saw me monthly. She was surprised and pleased she was able to stop Zoloft completely without any depressive recurrence, with the added bonus of less jitteriness and more enjoyable sexual intimacy. She continues to do well, but if and when she exhibits depressive symptoms again, I will restart Zoloft.

Measuring Change in Bipolar Disorders
Strategies for Increasing Stability

As with depression, treatment for bipolar disorders is more effective when we measure changes in mood across time. Use a valid, reliable tool of your choice for measuring change in order to recognize the early onset of depressive or manic symptoms, and avoid settling for partial effectiveness. Tools with good clinical utility for bipolar disorders include the QIDS or PHQ-9 for depressive episodes, the Altman Self-Rating Mania scale for (hypo)mania, and the Internal State Scale for both states (see Appendix A). The Mood Disorder Questionnaire (MDQ) is also valid for use with adolescents, but it may give false positives, especially if your client has untreated ADHD. Whatever measure you prefer, use it. Communicate your data with prescribers to increase their ability to make good decisions about medications.

In my practice, I also often use the client's identified early target symptoms of (hypo)mania and their mood diary to track their mood states. Mood charting is very effective at increasing stability because it provides an objective picture of how the client has been doing across time. When you go see your health care provider and they ask how you've been doing, your response is likely to reflect how you've been doing the past few days, or maybe even the past week. Yet, when I see clients with bipolar disorders, I need to know what the course of their illness has been like since our last visit. Have they had three weeks of paralyzing depression and are just feeling better over the past four days? Or have they had two hypomanic episodes followed by a week of depression each time, and are just recently feeling better? Or have they been stable and euthymic all along, and the past four days reflect their continued progress? Clients across each of these three scenarios are likely to respond to the question "How have you been doing?" with the same answer: "Okay." However, I can only provide excellent psychopharmacology if I know the full course of their illness since our last visit. That is where mood charting comes in.

This evidence-based, underutilized strategy is a simple chart that requires one checkmark a day to describe whether the client is feeling manic, euthymic, or depressed. Over the course of a month, it provides a literal picture of mood fluctuation. A sample two-week chart is provided here, and a monthly mood chart can be found in Appendix B. Some of my clients put this chart on their refrigerator or on their phone with an alarm to remind them to fill it out. Mood charting can track other symptoms as well—such as sleep, anxiety, and irritability—so it increases clients' internal awareness of their mood and energy. In turn, they are better able to recognize signs of early instability and can take proactive measures, such as practicing mindfulness, self-compassion, and CBT. It also helps me make better decisions about psychiatric medication.

In my practice, I have adapted the chart by also asking that clients put an "S" on days they experience any suicidality. Suicide is one of the leading causes of death in clients with bipolar disorders. Each year, 49 percent of people living with the disorder report having had suicidal thoughts, 26 percent develop a suicide plan, and 16 percent carry out the plan (Yatham et al., 2018). Be sure to stay current on evidence-based clinical strategies and interventions, and regularly ask about suicidality, even when you don't think it is an issue.

Sample Two-Week Mood Chart

	1	2	3	4	5	6	7	8	9	10	11	12	13	14
(Hypo)mania: Increased energy, racing thoughts														
Euthymic: Enjoying life, feeling good														
Depressed: Low energy, feeling sluggish														

Sleep is my other big measure of (hypo)mania—that is, whether the client needs little sleep without feeling exhausted the next several days or feels full of energy. It is impossible to stay euthymic and stable with bipolar disorders and no sleep. Ask about your client's sleep habits and get into the details. How many hours do they spend tossing and turning? When they awaken, what happens? Keep asking to get a picture of a full 24 hours. I write letters of accommodation for clients whose jobs require shift changes. They typically can manage two shifts, but expecting them to rotate between three shifts is a recipe for destabilization. Melatonin taken one to two hours prior to going to bed can help with shift changes, but clients with bipolar disorders may require more intensive medication for sleep/wake assistance, such as a bedtime dose of Seroquel (quetiapine).

Work with your client to identify their early symptoms of instability, and develop a written plan of action for when these symptoms occur. Doing so is proven to decrease the intensity and length of future episodes. A typical "re-set plan" might include specific ways your client can re-stabilize, such as increasing social support, engaging in calming or pleasurable activities, ensuring adequate sleep (a powerful one!), and using a PRN dose of medication (if it has been recommended by their prescriber). Being able to quickly recognize the early onset of instability and respond right away directly affects the efficacy of the plan. Time is of the essence when it comes to ensuring long-term stability. Waiting for an appointment with the prescriber to adjust the medication often means another episode of (hypo)mania or depression.

People with any chronic disease, including bipolar disorders, are healthier overall when they are able to give up the belief that their disorder is shameful or something to deny or ignore. That means integrating bipolar disorder into their sense of self, processing grief and loss, and recognizing the trauma resulting from years of the disease. When clients accept their diagnosis as part of who they are, it makes it easier for them to stay on medications that are lifelong, often a hassle, and

Case Example

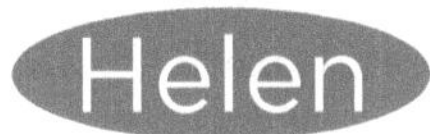

Helen, a 43-year-old woman with schizophrenia and bipolar I disorder, had been through 17 psychiatric hospitalizations, primarily for mania and psychosis. Her worst periods of depression always followed a manic episode, so she was highly motivated to stay stable. She had previously been on Seroquel (quetiapine), which did help stabilize her but resulted in unwanted weight gain.

Currently, she was taking the long-acting injectable Consta® (risperidone), which she felt was helpful, and Lamictal (lamotrigine), of which she wasn't so sure. She was also prescribed 1 mg tablets of Risperdal (risperidone) (up to two tablets daily) but only on an as-needed basis (PRN) for any "roughening" of symptoms.

When Helen came in for a recent medication check, she commented that she had experienced some symptoms of emerging mania about two weeks ago involving decreased need for sleep, racing thoughts, and excessive spending. She recognized the symptoms and took her PRN dose of Risperdal at bedtime for about five days. She also got some extra sleep, talked with her therapist that week, and returned "to being fine."

She smiled as she realized she had successfully managed her mania without an emergency room visit, hospitalization, or other disruption to her life for the first time. She continues to keep the bottle of Risperdal in her medicine cabinet "just in case."

commonly accompanied by several side effects. This is one strategy and avenue for strengthening stability that is routinely overlooked.

For some clients, though, the experience of long-term stability can cause them to feel a craving for the rush of mania and result in their discontinuing medication. It's as though the rhythm of bipolar cycling is deep in their cells, and when that cycling settles, they have an unconscious urge to feel it. Think of it like adults who grew up moving every few years who, now as adults, find themselves packing up to move "just because." I had one client who was psychiatrically hospitalized after discontinuing lithium when he had been stable on it for some time. When I asked him what happened, he shook his head and said, "I don't know. I didn't decide to, I just stopped taking it." Address this concern before it causes chaos for your client.

Ask Your Client

When your client is stable and feeling well, talk about the subconscious urge for increased energy as part of living with bipolar disorder. Predict the likelihood they will experience this urge and follow through with it. Articles in bp Magazine (the print edition) and bpHope (the online version) discuss this phenomenon and give suggestions. Written in a magazine format, the articles are approachable and normalize living with the disorder. One suggestion they provide involves using adrenaline-promoting activities to satisfy this almost cellular urge. You can also ask your client, "What might be some activities you could do to feel an adrenaline rush?" (Black diamond snowboarding, anyone?) Similarly, dbsalliance.org is an excellent resource for all things connected to mood disorders. Additional online and phone resources for supporting clients with bipolar disorders are available in Appendix B.

Vulnerable Populations

Pregnant Women

There is a high risk of recurrence of mood episodes during pregnancy, and there is no exception with bipolar disorders. Even for clients who are stable, 85 percent of women who discontinue their medication during pregnancy will become (hypo)manic or depressed, as will 37 percent of women who stay on their medication (Viguera et al., 2007). Not surprisingly, abruptly stopping medication during pregnancy is most likely to aggravate the situation, as most women will become (hypo)manic or depressed within two weeks.

When it comes to medications that are safe to take during pregnancy, lithium has less risk of birth defects than previously thought, so providers are increasingly recommending that women who are stable on this medication continue taking it during pregnancy (Wesseloo et al., 2017; Wieck, 2017). Lithium levels drop by 25 to 36 percent during the first and second trimester, so clients need regular blood draws. During the last six weeks of pregnancy, weekly blood draws are recommended. Postpartum lithium levels dramatically fluctuate as well, so levels should be checked twice weekly for the first two weeks following birth. Breastfeeding is not recommended when clients are on lithium due to risk of infant dehydration.

Although many atypical agents are often used in pregnancy, a recent study found that Risperdal (risperidone) has some incidence of birth defects and should be avoided (Huybrechts et al., 2015). Other atypical agents are considered reasonable options for treatment (Solmi et al., 2017). As discussed earlier, Depakote is contraindicated during pregnancy and for childbearing women in general, unless all other agents have failed. Interestingly, though, it is relatively safe to take when breastfeeding.

In general, women's health care providers are increasingly interested in the use of medication to keep clients with bipolar disorders stable and euthymic during pregnancy. (Hypo)mania and depression are harmful for the developing baby, as well as the mother. The best medication is usually the medication your client was on when she became pregnant. The fewer the agents the better. Additional up-to-date information on the recommended treatment options for women considering childbearing is available through womensmentalhealth.org.

Youth

Similar to depression, clients under the age of 25 manifest bipolar disorders differently than adults. When irritability is seen in youth, it is not a key symptom of bipolar disorders and is more likely reflective of underlying unipolar depression or anxiety. Similarly, severe mood dysregulation is also not indicative of bipolar disorders (Leibenluft, 2011). It is easy to mistakenly think an agitated, irritable young client has bipolar disorder when they really have depression.

Instead, look for grandiosity and increased goal-directed activity, which are more predictive of bipolar disorders. In youth, these symptoms can look like a change in energy with extreme or exaggerated plans for the future or for making money, and very high and unrealistic estimations of their personal abilities. Do not rely on family history (without symptoms) as a sole indicator, although mood disorders do have a high heritability rate. The incidence of major depressive disorder is so much more prevalent than bipolar disorders that you are likely to be wrong.

Assuming your client has a true diagnosis of bipolar disorder, youth are more sensitive to the adverse effects of medication. Therefore, dosages are started lower and gradually increased. Lower doses are generally equivalent to higher doses in effectiveness for youth but have more side effects. If your client is struggling with adverse effects, communicate this information to the prescriber right away, as they will likely slow down the titration rate or decrease the dosage. Do not assume your client will "get used to it." More than likely, they will just stop the medication.

With vulnerable clients, such as youth, I rely more heavily on agents that have a proven track record and save newer agents with less experience in clinical care as a last resort. For the treatment of acute mania in youth, lithium, Risperdal,

Abilify (aripiprazole), and Saphris (asenapine) are considered first-line treatments, whereas Latuda (lurasidone), lithium, and Lamictal (lamotrigine) are first-line in the treatment of acute depression. For the maintenance and prevention of these symptoms, lithium, Depakote (valproate), and Abilify are the preferred agents according to the CANMAT guidelines.

Lithium can be prescribed to children as young as 12, and most side effects in youth are similar to those in adults and can be managed similarly. Regularly measuring blood levels is just as important. Lithium does come in a liquid form, which is possibly useful for younger teens who struggle with swallowing pills. Its effectiveness does not "wear off," and its neuroprotective and anti-suicide effects are compelling. However, it can be dangerous on overdose.

In contrast to adults, Depakote is not indicated for the treatment of acute mania or depression in youth, though it is a top-tier agent for preventing these episodes and maintaining stability. However, it is not typically used for ongoing maintenance—especially among young women—because of its potential for weight gain, risk of polycystic ovarian syndrome, and serious teratogenicity concerns. Similar to adults, watch for sudden fatigue or confusion in young clients on Depakote; this can be a result of increased blood ammonia caused by the medication.

Lamictal is another effective agent for treating depressive episodes in youth with bipolar disorders, though it is not effective for treating or preventing mania. There is some evidence that it can also be used as a single-agent treatment for bipolar II disorder. Youth are prescribed a slightly lower dose than adults, which is usually in the range of 100-200 mg. However, the risk of Stevens-Johnson syndrome is higher in youth than adults, so alert your young client to this possibility and caution them not to increase Lamictal faster than prescribed. If your client discontinues or runs out of medication for more than a few days, they will likely need to restart the titration process from the beginning.

Remember, anticonvulsants such as Depakote and Lamictal have a black box warning for increased risk of suicidality. However, other anticonvulsants—such as Tegretol (carbamazepine) and Trileptal (oxcarbazepine)—are not recommended agents for youth due to their lack of effectiveness.

Finally, while atypical agents (e.g., Risperdal, Abilify, Saphris, Latuda) are commonly used to treat bipolar disorders in youth, they do have serious adverse effects. Youth are extremely sensitive to the weight gain from these agents, and a 30-pound weight gain in two weeks in not unusual with certain medications.

Older Adults

Generally, older adults have lived with their bipolar disorder for decades. They have had experience with many medications, know what works and doesn't work, and understand what causes adverse effects. Spending some time getting to know this history is very helpful. Bipolar disorders rarely occur with a first episode after 50, so if an older client is presenting with what looks like (hypo)mania, contact their primary care provider right away. It is highly likely these symptoms reflect delirium or another medical condition.

Case Example

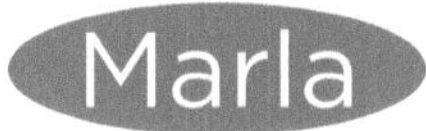

Marla, a 72-year-old woman with bipolar disorder, had done very well the past several years on a combination of Lamictal (lamotrigine) and Latuda (lurasidone). Over the past year, though, she complained more about her memory. It continued to worsen, and a screening test using the Montreal Cognitive Assessment showed that she had deteriorated to the dementia range of functioning.

Her primary care provider ordered lab and imaging tests to rule out other causes. Because of her age and the fact that anticonvulsants are known to cause a wide variety of adverse effects, I started decreasing her Lamictal, and over the next few weeks, she noticed an improved ability to remember things.

We continued to decrease the dose gradually without any recurrence of depressive symptoms, and her memory continued to improve. She now is on a very low dose of Lamictal (50 mg), her mood has remained stable, and she scores in the normal range of cognitive functioning. Sometimes, deprescribing is the best prescribing, especially for older adults.

In addition, older adults with bipolar disorders tend to have progressively less intense episodes of (hypo)mania. Instead, they are more likely to experience predominant depressive episodes and can be frequently misdiagnosed as having major depressive disorder (which then leads to inappropriate treatment). The importance of accurate treatment cannot be understated, as lifelong, poorly treated or untreated mood disorders are associated with poorer cognitive functioning and earlier cognitive decline (James et al., 2018).

The three recommended top-line agents for the treatment of bipolar disorders in older adults are lithium, Lamictal, and Depakote. When lithium is used, older adults tend to do well with slightly lower levels (0.4-0.6 mEq/l), and for those over the age of 80, the maximum level is 0.7 mEq/l. Additionally, the dose needed to get a therapeutic level decreases with age. For example, clients in their eighties require approximately 30 percent of the dose they needed in their thirties (Rej et al., 2014). Depakote dosing is not as affected by aging, and the required dose may remain similar to what worked and provided a therapeutic blood level in younger years.

Seroquel (quetiapine) is a second-tier medication used for the treatment of bipolar disorders in older adults, and it is the best of the atypical agents for this population. The other atypicals are not commonly used because these medications are associated with a very high rate of movements disorders, such as dystonia and tardive dyskinesia (see Chapter 4). Although medications like Cogentin® (benztropine) are used to treat movement disorders caused by atypical agents, they also have a heavy anticholinergic burden that can worsen cognitive impairment in older adults. Because Seroquel has a low potential to cause movement disorders, it is the preferred choice of the atypicals. Unfortunately, it can wreak havoc on blood sugar levels, which can be problematic for those with diabetes.

Across all classes of medications, lower doses may be needed when treating older adults to avoid sedation or cognitive impairment, though older adults tend not to be so vulnerable to akathisia. Benzodiazepines are not recommended in older adults, even as an add-on to other mood stabilizers, because of its associated risk of falls and memory impairment (see Chapter 5 for more information on benzodiazepines).

Co-occurring Substance Use Disorders

Making an accurate diagnosis of bipolar disorder can be challenging with clients with substance use disorders. For example, the use of methamphetamine can look like mania (or schizophrenia). Similarly, when clients are in the early stages of recovery, post-acute withdrawal syndrome (PAWS) can look like bipolar disorder, as it also presents with rapidly changing moods, irritability, and sleep disturbance. One symptom of PAWS, difficulty with balance, helps to differentiate it from bipolar disorders. Therefore, getting a good longitudinal history is helpful. Were there times when your client was clean and sober for a significant period (over six months) and met criteria for (hypo)mania? If not, be very cautious about the diagnosis.

Clients with comorbid substance use and bipolar disorders have specific complications that inform treatment decisions when it comes to medication. For example, clients who engage in intravenous drug use often have difficulty with blood draws and are thus poor candidates for lithium. They may stop the dose, and lithium is not a good agent to frequently discontinue and restart. It stops working and causes a rebound in mania or suicidality when suddenly stopped. If your client is likely to stop their medication when using substances, lithium is not recommended.

Clients with substance use disorders tend to do well on agents that are slightly more sedating, such as some atypical antipsychotics and Depakote. While Depakote also requires blood draws, there is more latitude than with lithium. If blood cell production and liver functioning are well within the normal range, then prescribers will often check blood levels less frequently. I have also found that clients prefer taking part of their Depakote dose during the day, as it has a slight anti-anxiety effect, and the remaining majority of the dose at bedtime to help them sleep. Provided there are no contraindications, such as having cirrhosis of the liver, having had pancreatitis, or being a woman of childbearing capacity, Depakote can be a very effective agent.

Clients with alcohol use disorders are more likely to have liver disease, which may preclude use of Depakote. Depakote is "hepatotoxic," meaning that it is stressful on the liver. For those clients, lithium may be a better choice. It does not affect the liver and is directly excreted by the kidneys.

Atypical agents can also be very effective, although I avoid or very slowly titrate agents that cause more akathisia, such as Abilify. Clients with co-occurring substance use disorders tend to be very sensitive to akathisia and will simply stop their medication. In addition, many clients with a history of substance use—who are now in recovery—began using drugs in the first place in an attempt to avoid these similar feelings of psychomotor anxiety. In this case, the use of atypicals can actually trigger relapse in an effort to alleviate the restless and jittery feelings.

Be sure to educate your client about the importance of continuing to take their psychotropic medication even if they use substances. I tell my clients that's when their brain needs it the very most. The only exception to this "rule" involves benzodiazepines, which should not be prescribed to individuals actively using substances. In the rare circumstances when benzodiazepines are prescribed, they should not be taken when your client uses any sedating substances, such as opiates or alcohol.

For clients with co-occurring substance use disorders, treating their bipolar disorder is critical to their long-term recovery. Oftentimes, mood swings are the triggers for relapse or increased use, so helping them achieve stability is key.

Conclusion

We have so much room for improvement in helping clients with bipolar disorders experience less suffering and achieve more joy and satisfaction in life. You are an important motivator, coach, safety net, and observer of change in this process. Ask questions, assess for suicidality, and review mood charts in your session. In addition, talk with their prescriber by communicating your observations of change (both in terms of improvement and roughening of stability) and voicing your concerns. There are few places in the mental health field where we have more potential to make such a huge difference than we do in the treatment of bipolar disorders.

Treatment of Psychosis and Other Uses of Atypical Antipsychotics

The treatment of psychosis, including schizophrenia and other psychotic-spectrum disorders, involves medication to reduce the frequency and intensity of hallucinations, delusions, and paranoia—as well as the fears that result from these "brain tricks." Medications are less helpful with treating the so-called negative symptoms, which include low motivation, poverty of speech, blunted affect, and cognitive impairments (e.g., deficits in processing speed, memory, and executive function). Individuals with psychotic disorders often, but not always, require lifelong medication to manage their symptoms, though older adults may need less medication as the intensity of their symptoms wane in later decades.

Like all illnesses, the psychotic disorders vary in severity and chronicity, but they are typically on the more disabling end. The severity of these disorders makes it easy to forget that clients with psychosis are far more different from one another than they are similar. And recovery from psychosis—that is, less time spent suffering, fewer hospitalizations, and being able to experience more satisfaction, joy, and meaning in life—happens with the right medications, psychotherapies, and social supports.

In this chapter, I will describe the differences and similarities between typical and atypical antipsychotics, and under what circumstances they are useful. I will provide specific questions you can ask your client to assess for potential problems associated with the use of these medications, including how to recognize serious side effects, and discuss ways to measure change. I'll also give you effective strategies to decrease the fear and stigma associated with taking antipsychotics and discuss how to motivate clients to consider taking medication or continue with their current medication when it is working. This chapter includes both the science of medication and the art of helping clients find a good medication choice and take it consistently. Finally, I'll highlight the use of antipsychotics with vulnerable populations, especially in light of the growing role and prevalence of atypical antipsychotics.

Typical vs. Atypical Antipsychotics

There are two classes of antipsychotic medication, which are commonly referred to as the "typical" and "atypical" antipsychotics. Typical antipsychotics tend to be older agents, and their usage is predominantly for treating psychosis. Atypical antipsychotics tend to be newer, and in addition to treating psychosis, they treat other non-psychotic conditions. However, this difference is not what makes a medication typical or atypical.

Rather, what differentiates these two classes of medications is the percentage of dopamine post-receptor sites that they block. All antipsychotics affect the neurotransmitter dopamine, but to different degrees. When less than 65 percent of post-receptor sites are blocked, you get no antipsychotic benefit. When over 80 percent are blocked, the brain floods with dopamine—even into unwanted pathways—which often results in abnormal, involuntary movements (e.g., swaying or jerking patterns) and hormonal side effects (e.g., increases in prolactin levels resulting in hyperprolactinemia). These effects are seen with the typical antipsychotics, such as Haldol® (haloperidol), Prolixin® (fluphenazine), and many others.

In contrast, atypical medications block between 65 and 80 percent of the dopamine receptor sites, which is a "sweet spot" of sorts. These medications provide antipsychotic benefit without the extensive abnormal movements or hormonal side effects seen with typical agents. They also effectively treat a wide range of conditions in addition to psychosis, such as bipolar disorders and autism spectrum disorders.

Typical Antipsychotics

Typical agents, which are sometimes referred to as first-generation antipsychotics, are effective in the treatment of psychotic disorders, regardless of the underlying cause of the psychosis. For example, they work for schizophrenia, drug-induced psychosis, and psychosis in acute mania. Haldol (haloperidol) is also used to treat Tourette's disorder, a neurological tic disorder. However, these agents are not effective for the treatment of bipolar disorders, with the exception of the acute treatment of mania, because they do not provide a "stabilizing" effect over time.

Given that typical agents were initially developed in the 1950s, you may have clients who have been taking them for years or even decades. These agents tend to be less expensive than the atypicals, and they also do not adversely affect blood sugar (glucose) or cholesterol and triglycerides (lipids). Therefore, they can be a good choice for clients with diabetes or hyperlipidemia. Some of the common typical agents are listed in the following table.

Commonly Used Typical Antipsychotics

Brand Name	Generic Name	Dosage Range	Comments
Thorazine® (was)	Chlorpromazine	50-600 mg	Can cause photosensitivity
Prolixin	Fluphenazine	2-20 mg	Long-acting injectable available
Haldol	Haloperidol	2-20 mg	Long-acting injectable available
Trilafon® (was)	Perphenazine	8-64 mg	
Mellaril® (was)	Thioridazine	5-600 mg	Can cause cardiac rhythm changes involving QTc prolongation
Navane®	Thiothixene	6-40 mg	
Stelazine® (was)	Trifluoperazine	4-40 mg	

However, the use of typical antipsychotics has declined over the years because of their potential to cause extrapyramidal symptoms. These symptoms include akathisia, dystonia, and pseudoparkinsonism—as well as tardive dyskinesia, which is a long-term and sometimes permanent movement disorder.

In contrast to the akathisia often associated with the use of SSRIs, the akathisia resulting from typical antipsychotics is far more pronounced. Akathisia on antipsychotics feels like, perhaps, drinking 40 cups of coffee. It literally becomes impossible to sit still. You will see clients pacing, wringing their hands, shaking their legs, and talking about their skin "crawling." They will be unable to sit calmly in your office. The symptoms tend to begin hours to days after starting the medication.

Historically, clients with serious akathisia sought treatment at emergency rooms because of their distress, where they would often be misdiagnosed as agitated or psychotic—and, of course, be given more of the offending antipsychotic, often Haldol, which only served to increase the akathisia. Fortunately, urgent care settings have gotten better at making this differential diagnosis and providing effective treatment. The first-line treatment for akathisia is propranolol or benzodiazepines. If those don't work, other medications to consider include Symmetrel® (amantadine), Remeron (mirtazapine), and clonidine. Cogentin (benztropine) can also be tried, though it often has little effect on akathisia.

In addition to akathisia, typical antipsychotics can cause dystonia, pseudoparkinsonism, and other types of rigidity and tightness in the muscles. Dystonia involves an involuntary and uncomfortable (often painful) tightening or cramping of the muscles, frequently in the arms, legs, or jaw. Pseudoparkinsonism causes rigidity in how your client walks, sits, and holds their body. However, clients may not connect these symptoms to the antipsychotic medication since this adverse effect can creep in and occur days, weeks, or even months after starting the medication.

There are several medications that are effective for treating dystonia and pseudoparkinsonism, including Cogentin, Benadryl® (diphenhydramine), Symmetrel (amantadine), and Artane® (trihexyphenidyl). However, Artane is used infrequently because of its tendency toward agitation, and its hallucinogenic properties can result in the potential for abuse at high doses. The next table includes a list of medications used to treat the adverse movement effects often caused by typical antipsychotics.

Abnormal Movement Medications

Brand Name	Generic Name	Use	Dose	Comments
Inderal®	Propranolol	Akathisia	10-20 mg twice daily	Dose may be less or greater
Artane	Trihexyphenidyl	Dystonia, rigidity	5-10 mg	Potential for abuse
Benadryl	Diphenhydramine	Dystonia, rigidity, eyes rolling back (oculogyric crisis)	25-100 mg	Comes in a long-acting injectable formulation
Cogentin	Benztropine	Dystonia, rigidity, akathisia (small effect)	0.5-4 mg	Heavy anticholinergic burden
Symmetrel	Amantadine	Dystonia, akathisia	100-200 mg	Less anticholinergic burden
Austedo®	Deutetrabenazine	Tardive dyskinesia	12-48 mg	Requires a 2-month titration period
Ingrezza®	Valbenazine	Tardive dyskinesia	40-80 mg	
Klonopin	Clonazepam	Tardive dyskinesia	0.5-1 mg	Very limited evidence
Catapres®	Clonidine	Akathisia	0.2 mg	Second-line agent
Remeron	Mirtazipine	Akathisia	15 mg	Second-line agent

Ask Your Client

Take extrapyramidal symptoms seriously. Ask about restlessness, tightness, cramping, and stiffness. These conditions are very uncomfortable and are a common reason your clients will stop taking their medication. This is especially true if they feel their concerns and complaints are being minimized or ignored, so take the time to ask details. What exactly are the symptoms like? Are the symptoms worse at certain times of day? Do they notice the symptoms more when they are still or moving? Do others notice? I also tend to ask about tightness in the jaw or teeth grinding in particular because clients may have chronic back pain that I don't want to confuse with dystonia.

Communicate your observations with the prescriber and explain the specific symptoms your client has described. Make sure to include a specific question in your message to clarify whether the prescriber would like the client to come in right away, or whether they'd like to change the medication dose or start a different medication altogether. Include your client's pharmacy information in case the prescriber wants to send in a new prescription.

Finally, tardive dyskinesia is an abnormal movement disorder caused by typical antipsychotics, though it can be caused by one of the atypicals as well (Risperdal, or risperidone). It is characterized by involuntary, purposeless, repetitive, rolling-type movements that primarily affect the tongue and mouth, facial muscles, and extremities. This is "the look" of schizophrenia. Although these movements are not acutely painful, they are annoying and can become permanent. The movements can also be disfiguring. One client of mine likened it to having leprosy as he described the embarrassment and ostracization he experienced when strangers took two steps away on the commuter train after seeing him. Older adults are extremely vulnerable to tardive dyskinesia, as are clients who have been on typical agents for many years.

There are now medications that treat tardive dyskinesia, including Ingrezza (valbenazine) and Austedo (deutetrabenazine). These medications are effective, even when the client has had tardive dyskinesia for years. They are also non-addicting. However, they are not suitable for clients on methadone or who have a prolonged QTc in their heart rhythm, so clients should have an EKG prior to treatment. Although these medications are extremely expensive, they do have patient assistance programs. Some insurance companies first require a trial of Klonopin (clonazepam) to cover these medications, except when the client has a history of addiction to benzodiazepines.

It is definitely worth having a conversation with your client about medications that treat these movement disorders. You may be the catalyst to encourage your client to ask their prescriber about extrapyramidal symptoms and how these medications can help. The Abnormal Involuntary Movement Scale (AIMS) is the tool of choice to measure and monitor change in tardive dyskinesia (see Appendix A). It is standard care to screen for and track tardive dyskinesia by prescribers, although it is not always done.

In addition to movement disorders, the typical antipsychotics are also associated with hormonal side effects. In particular, these medications can result in elevated prolactin levels, a condition known as hyperprolactinemia, which results in enhanced breast development or actual breast secretions (called galactorrhea)—even among males. Elevated prolactin also increases the desire to stay home and "nest," which is evolutionarily helpful for breastfeeding mothers, but not for a 27-year-old client trying to recover from a first episode of psychosis. It also causes depression in men and increases the risk of fractures on falls.

Finally, typical antipsychotics likely exacerbate paucity of thought and the expressionless, almost rigid, facial expression experienced by many individuals with psychosis. These negative symptoms of psychosis are very disabling. Atypical agents seem to have less of this adverse effect.

Atypical Antipsychotics

The newer generation of antipsychotic medications, known as atypical antipsychotics, are equally as effective as the typical antipsychotics in treating psychosis. In fact, one atypical agent, Clozaril® (clozapine), is a more effective than all others. However, atypicals also do more than treat psychosis, which is why they are frequently referred to as atypical "agents," and they are very effective mood stabilizers, even for clients without psychosis. In particular, they are also effective in treating mania, depressive episodes, and for ensuring "maintenance"—that is, the prevention of future mood episodes in bipolar disorders. This mood stabilization effect reflects a separate action from its effect on psychosis. The Atypical Antipsychotics table provides a list of these atypical medications, which include Risperdal (risperidone), Seroquel (quetiapine), Zyprexa (olanzapine), Abilify (aripiprazole), Geodon® (ziprasidone), Latuda (lurasidone), Fanapt® (iloperidone), Invega (paliperidone), and Clozaril, among others.

Atypical Antipsychotics

Brand Name	Generic Name	Dosage Range	Comments
Abilify	Aripiprazole	5-30 mg	Most prone to cause akathisia; Long-acting injectable available
Saphris	Asenapine	5-20 mg at bedtime	Must be dissolved and absorbed under the tongue (avoiding food or drink for 10 minutes after); Has a bitter taste
Rexulti®	Brexpiprazole	1-4 mg	Associated with more akathisia
Vraylar	Cariprazine	1.5-6 mg	Can possibly assist with the cognitive symptoms of schizophrenia

Clozaril	Clozapine	12.5-900 mg	Most effective antipsychotic; Only used for treatment-resistant schizophrenia
Fanapt	Iloperidone	2-24 mg	Causes problematic dizziness and must be increased gradually
Latuda	Lurasidone	40-160 mg	Must been taken with 350 kcal of food; Very low incidence of akathisia and dystonia
Zyprexa	Olanzapine	5-20 mg	Available in oral and dissolvable tablet form; Long-acting injectable also available, but with significant limitations
Invega	Paliperidone	6-12 mg	Long-acting injectable available
Nuplazid®	Pimavanserin	34 mg	Only used for psychosis in Parkinson's disease
Seroquel	Quetiapine	50- 800 mg	Causes the least amount of akathisia and dystonia; Most sedating
Risperdal	Risperidone	1-8 mg	Long-acting injectable available
Geodon	Ziprasidone	20-160 mg	Must be taken with 500 kcal of food; Affects QTc (heart rhythm)

In addition, atypical agents can be used to augment antidepressants in major depressive disorder and are even considered first-line in the treatment of major depressive disorder with "mixed" features, such as mood lability, irritability, and racing thoughts. Atypical agents are the medication of choice for treating anorexia nervosa, and they are effective in treating the psychosis seen in severe PTSD and OCD. These agents are also effective in decreasing the intensity of the angst experienced by clients with borderline personality disorder and are effective in treatment-resistant anxiety disorders. However, the atypical agents act in an adjunctive, supporting capacity for the treatment of these conditions, as psychotherapy is still considered the gold-standard treatment option. Finally, atypical agents treat the agitation associated with autism spectrum disorders and dementia, though there are significant risks to using atypical agents for clients with dementia (see Vulnerable Populations section).

Alert Your Client

Be certain to reassure your client that taking an atypical agent for another condition, such as bipolar disorder, does not mean they are psychotic or have schizophrenia. The mood stabilization effect of the atypicals represents a completely separate and additional use of this class of medication.
The pharmacist may inform clients that these medications are used for the treatment of psychosis and schizophrenia, so if you haven't had this conversation with your clients ahead of time, clients will likely throw away their medication or refuse it at the pharmacy.

The atypical agents really are multi-use medications, but they do have potential side effects as well. While these medications are usually associated with a reduced incidence of extrapyramidal symptoms, they can still cause both akathisia and dystonia. In addition, they have more problems with weight gain and metabolic issues.

Weight gain can occur with all antipsychotics, but some of the atypical agents can cause serious, significant weight gain, such as 10 or 20 pounds in a month—and if left unchecked, even 70 pounds or greater. Some of the agents that are more likely to cause weight gain include Zyprexa, Seroquel, and Risperdal. Not all clients gain weight, though, even on agents that are prone to cause weight gain. It is highly individual.

In addition, the atypical agents cause adverse metabolic effects involving increased blood sugar (glucose) that can lead to diabetes, as well as increased cholesterol and triglycerides (lipids) that can lead to stroke and other cardiovascular events. These adverse effects vary between the atypical agents and between clients (see following table). Some clients have trouble with these metabolic effects, while others do not. Unfortunately, there is no way to predict which of your clients will have problems. These metabolic changes do not occur with the typical antipsychotics.

Increased abdominal girth is the best indicator of underlying metabolic problems while clients are taking these medications, so if your client notices abdominal weight gain, they absolutely need to see their prescribing provider. However, even clients who do not gain weight on these medications can still experience adverse impacts on their blood glucose or lipids. Therefore, they will need to get their blood drawn several times a year.

Determination of metabolic risk is based on population data, which provides us with an estimate of how likely adverse effects are to happen. Because these are population estimates, even a medication with a lower incidence rate might cause problems for your client. Conversely, a medication considered high risk may cause them no problems at all. For example, Zyprexa is considered high risk because more people have been found to develop problems on it compared to the percentage of those on Geodon. However, I have more than a dozen clients who have done well on Zyprexa without gaining a pound and whose blood glucose and cholesterol levels are normal. At the same time, I've also had many more clients I've had to take off Zyprexa due to weight gain and metabolic problems.

Population-Based Risk of Metabolic Adversity

	Low	Medium	Medium-High	High
Risk of Metabolic Adversity	Abilify, Latuda, Geodon	Saphris, Rexulti, Vraylar, Fanapt	Invega, Seroquel, Risperdal	Clozaril, Zyprexa

The good news is that these problems can be minimized by changing the medication to one with less metabolic adversity. For example, if your client has gained

30 pounds while taking Risperdal and they lose 20 pounds after being switched to Geodon, Latuda, or Vraylar, then their blood glucose levels may normalize. It also helps to stop or decrease the consumption of sugary beverages. Soda, energy drinks, and other sweetened beverages can significantly worsen weight gain and cause increases in glucose levels. I had one client who kept gaining weight until his primary care provider finally determined he was drinking a gallon of chocolate milk every day. I hadn't thought to ask about that when reviewing his diet.

Because metabolic adversity can pose serious health concerns, it is critical that clients monitor their blood about twice yearly when taking these medications. Clients may need to increase the frequency of these blood checks if there are creeping metabolic and weight issues, or they may require these checks less frequently if there has been a long period of stability with no changes.

Changes in blood glucose are monitored by a hemoglobin A1c test, which gives a picture of the blood glucose levels over the past several months, not just at the time of the blood draw. It indicates whether a client's levels are normal, pre-diabetic, or diabetic. If your client moves from normal to pre-diabetic, encourage them to talk with their prescribing provider about options, including changing to a medication with less metabolic risk or starting Metformin. Metformin can effectively prevent and minimize weight gain and metabolic problems due to atypical agents, and clients are less likely to progress toward diabetes on this medication. It is most effective when started early rather than after your client has gained substantial weight.

Encourage your clients to track their weight and be proactive. Early detection can prevent serious weight gain with significant medical consequences. In addition, have a conversation about your client's unique eating and drinking habits, and their amount of daily movement.

Ask Your Client

Unfortunately, not all prescribing providers watch and monitor for metabolic concerns. Be sure your client gets their blood glucose levels monitored on a regular basis by explicitly asking, "When was the last time you had your blood sugar checked?" If it was more than six months ago, alert the prescriber and ask if the client should make an appointment to see them first or go directly to the lab for testing.

The Specific Agents

Because the atypical agents are quite different from each other in terms of their side effects and specific instructions regarding how to take them, I'll review them individually. However, it is worth noting that with the exception of Fanapt, all these agents can be taken once a day, which increases their potential for success. Think of twice-daily dosing as doubling the risk your client will not get the amount needed for effectiveness. It increases the chance your client will miss doses of medication or

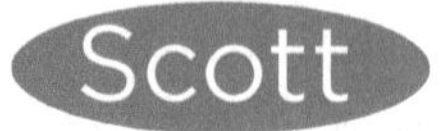

Scott was a 52-year-old man with a history of multiple addictions, though he had been clean and sober for 10 years. He had suffered with lifelong depressive episodes and been on many antidepressants with some brief, limited response. When he came to see me, he had been staying in bed—according to his partner's report—for weeks, maybe months. His partner was becoming distraught over Scott's worsening withdrawal and agitation with her. Scott was still taking 40 mg of Prozac (fluoxetine), which he had thought was working when I saw him about three months earlier. Now he presented as gaunt and endorsed experiencing both hopelessness and suicidal ideation. He didn't want to die, but he felt so frustrated by his depression that he didn't know what else to do. His PHQ-9 score was 24. He also reported having persistent, racing thoughts, which he said were "driving me nuts." He was easily irritated, as I saw in the interview, almost in spite of himself.

Scott had never had a hypomanic or manic episode, nor did he meet the criteria for any of the bipolar disorders. Based on his symptom presentation, it was clear he had major depressive disorder with mixed features, or what in previous decades might have been called an agitated depression. I stopped Prozac and started him on a trial of Abilify (aripiprazole) after reviewing medication options and discussing their likely benefits and risks. A week or two later I received a message in the electronic health record from Scott's primary care provider thanking me. Scott had come in wanting to get his poorly controlled asthma under control and asked for help to stop smoking.

When I saw him shortly after, Scott was well-groomed, smiling, and amazed at how much better he felt. Needless to say, his partner was also very pleased. His PHQ-9 score had dropped to 14. Fortunately, he tolerated the Abilify well without side effects. He continues to do well on Abilify, and his PHQ-9 score is now in the non-depressed range, with no further depressive episodes over the past year.

discontinue their medication altogether, leading to worsened symptoms and increased hospitalization rates (Brown & Bussell, 2011; Morken, Widen, & Grawe, 2008). So make sure to ask about their medication: what they like and don't like, the hassles of taking it, and what helps them in the process. You may be surprised.

Abilify

Abilify is an effective atypical agent used for the treatment of schizophrenia, and it is also used for treating and preventing mania in bipolar disorders, for augmenting antidepressants in treatment-resistant depression, for easing symptoms of irritability in autism, and for treating tics in Tourette's syndrome. It is also the initial medication of choice for major depressive disorder with mixed features.

Abilify is one of the more energizing atypical agents, so many clients like taking it in the morning. Some clients experience that energizing side effect as anxiety, so be sure to ask about this. It also has a high incidence of akathisia. Once in a while I have a client who prefers taking it at bedtime because it makes them sleepy. Uncommonly, it can trigger uncontrollable gambling and other impulse control problems, such as compulsive shopping or sexual behaviors. The medication needs to be stopped in these situations.

Once-a-day dosing is effective and much easier for most people to maintain, especially for conditions requiring long-term treatment. Aripiprazole is also available in a monthly long-acting injectable called Maintena®, which is well-tolerated and increases stability in schizophrenia and bipolar disorders (see section on Using Long-Acting Injectables).

Clozaril

Clozaril treats psychosis better than any other medication and is considered the gold standard of treatment for schizophrenia. However, it is prescribed only for clients who have failed on other agents because, although it works very well, it has significant side effects and potential dangers. In particular, it can cause changes in blood cell production (agranulocytosis) that can be fatal.

The potential for these adverse effects resulted in Clozaril being taken off the market in the U.S. shortly after it was introduced in the 1970s, though it was reintroduced in the 1990s with very strict monitoring requirements for safety. Clients who start Clozaril must get their blood drawn weekly and have those lab results sent to the pharmacy, which is then allowed to dispense one week of medication. No lab results, no medication. This process occurs every week for the first six months. If no abnormalities occur, the frequency of blood draws drops to every other week for another six months. Again, if no abnormalities are present, blood draws drop to monthly for as long as clients take the medication.

Clozaril also has many other challenges, such as weight gain, increases in blood glucose and lipids, cardiac problems, drooling, and over-sedation, to name a few. In spite of these side challenges, this medication is unparalleled when it comes to eliminating psychotic symptoms that have been plaguing clients for years or even decades without relief. It allows individuals who have been previously unable to function to live independently and enjoy life. In Europe, they tend to use Clozaril more often and, not coincidentally, have better outcomes in clients with schizophrenia.

Fanapt

Fanapt is a less commonly used atypical that is indicated for the treatment of schizophrenia. In practice, it is also used for treating bipolar disorders, augmenting antidepressants in major depression, and managing impulse control disorders. It is a more challenging atypical in that it is the one exception to once-daily dosing and must be taken twice daily. Fanapt can also cause heart rhythm changes involving QTc prolongation, so it is not a good medication for clients on methadone or those with serious liver disease.

Fanapt also requires gradually increasing the dose to avoid orthostatic hypotension (e.g., low blood pressure upon standing up). If your client has been off Fanapt for more than three days, they will need to restart the titration process all over again to reduce the symptoms of dizziness associated with starting this medication. Because of these side effects, this agent is generally reserved for use when others have failed or are not tolerated.

Geodon

Geodon is indicated for treatment of schizophrenia and bipolar disorders, and it also comes in an immediate-action injectable often used in emergency departments for agitation associated with schizophrenia. However, it is not listed as a top-tier medication in the CANMAT review because some studies have shown that it does not work in the treatment of acute mania or depression, and it works only in combination with lithium or Depakote (valproate) for maintenance (Yatham et al., 2018).

Geodon works best when taken with 500 kcal of food, as up to 50 percent of the dose never gets absorbed if taken on an empty stomach. However, expecting your client to take this medication twice daily and with 500 kcal of food at each dose is unrealistic. It is better to decide on a meal where they routinely eat more than 500 kcal and take the full daily dose then. Because of its food requirement, Geodon is not a good choice for clients living in institutions where food and "med time" are hours apart, such as jails, prison, and possibly nursing homes. Ask your client what works best for them. I have some clients who have a pattern of munching all day long and never eat 500 kcal at one time, so I choose an alternative medication.

Like Fanapt, Geodon also can also cause QTc prolongation, which can become dangerous if your client is taking methadone or certain other medications, including tricyclic antidepressants. It also tends to be activating, although it is not associated with the akathisia seen with Abilify. Of the atypicals, it has perhaps the least amount of weight gain and metabolic problems. However, Geodon tends to be under-prescribed because the original FDA dosing guidelines, which were based on short-term trials with very narrow inclusion criteria, recommend a lower dosage than that which is commonly required. This low dosing may also have contributed to studies finding it less effective.

Latuda

Latuda has demonstrated particular effectiveness in treating clients with bipolar disorders, notably those with depressive episodes, and it is a second-tier medication in maintaining stability. It is less sedating and is well tolerated by many clients. Weight gain can happen, as can metabolic problems, but they're not common. It is an excellent medication option for clients who don't like feeling sedated or have suffered significant depressive episodes in bipolar disorders. It works best in combination with lithium or Depakote for bipolar depression.

Similar to Geodon, Latuda must be taken with food in order to be fully absorbed, though the caloric requirement is slightly less (350 kcal). It does not need to be taken twice daily, and the full daily dose can be taken with any meal, which significantly increases its effectiveness as a long-term medication. Although it is expensive, many insurance companies will cover this medication quite readily once they are assured it isn't the first atypical to have been prescribed. Perhaps the decreased cost of rehospitalization outweighs the cost of this medication.

Ask Your Client

Many clients do not have an accurate sense of what 350 kcal is. Ask your client when they take their medication and if they eat at that time. I had one client who was eating an additional full dinner at 10 p.m. with his Latuda (lurasidone), which helped with medication absorption, but also caused significant weight gain. It is helpful to provide your client with a cheat sheet of 350 kcal food ideas, making sure to include both healthy and convenient options. A sample food guide is provided in Appendix B. Because Latuda is not particularly sedating, I encourage my clients to try taking their medication after dinner rather than at bedtime.

Risperdal

Risperdal was one of the first atypical agents available, and many insurance companies require that clients try this medication before agreeing to pay for the more expensive, newer medications. Risperdal is an unusual agent in that at low doses it functions as an atypical by blocking between 65 to 80 percent of dopamine post-receptor sites. However, at higher doses (about 3+ mg) it becomes a typical antipsychotic and is associated with an accompanying increase in akathisia, dystonia, and tardive dyskinesia. Similar to typical antipsychotics, it can also increase prolactin at higher doses (hyperprolactinemia). Therefore, if you are working with a client who takes Risperdal and you notice any difference in side effects, ask if they have had a recent increase in dose. If so, connect your client with their prescriber to either change the medication or address the side effects. Remember, clients tend to stop medication that is uncomfortable.

Risperidone comes in a long-acting injectable form called Consta, which is given every two weeks, as well as a newer formulation that is monthly but trickier to administer. Recent studies have also found that Risperdal is associated with adverse fetal outcomes (Damkler, 2018), so it is now the last atypical prescribed to women of childbearing capacity or who are pregnant.

Invega

Invega is related to Risperdal and has many of the same side effects, although it may cause less weight gain and is not associated with hyperprolactinemia. Invega comes in multiple long-acting injectable formulations that require monthly (or tri-monthly) injections (compared to risperidone, which requires bi-weekly injections). It can be sedating, although some clients experience it as calming. It is a top-tier medication for the treatment of schizophrenia and acute mania in bipolar disorders, and it is also effective for maintaining stability in bipolar disorders. It does not need to be taken with food and is less sedating than Risperdal.

Seroquel

Seroquel is an atypical agent that is effective in treating psychosis, augmenting antidepressant medications, and both preventing and treating manic and depressive symptoms in bipolar disorders. The range for effective dosing is wide, as some clients do well on 100 to 200 mg daily, while others need up to 800 mg to effectively treat schizophrenia. For clients with bipolar disorders, studies show its effectiveness does not increase beyond 300 mg, although individual clients may experience it differently.

Because it is probably the most sedating antipsychotic, it was—and still is, although hopefully less so—used as a sleep aid for the general population. This practice has been discouraged because the risks of weight gain and metabolic adversity far outweighs the benefits. Many other agents can help you sleep. Its sedating effect is not linear, as it doesn't get progressively more sedating as the dose is increased. Rather, the sedation plateaus around 200 mg.

In addition, Seroquel can cause hypotension if the dose is not gradually increased over several days. The extended-release version does not cause this problem, but it also does not have the same immediate sedating effect that provides the sleep assistance many people like. If your clients are using the extended-release version, they may find that it works better to take Seroquel a few hours before bed.

Zyprexa

Zyprexa is another atypical agent that can effectively treat psychosis and mania. However, it is considered a high-risk medication due to its potential to cause weight gain and an increase in blood glucose and lipids. Although not everyone will experience these problems, individuals on Zyprexa require vigilant monitoring to assess for signs of metabolic adversity. On the other hand, it tends not to cause as much akathisia as some of the other antipsychotics. It is sedating, so many clients prefer taking it at bedtime. Once-daily dosing is effective. It does not matter if it is taken with or without food. Zyprexa can also be very useful as a PRN "rescue med" in the treatment of acute manic or psychosis. In these situations, clients can take a full therapeutic dose—for example, 15 mg—without needing to gradually increase over several days.

Using Long-Acting Injectables

One of the significant ways to help increase stability and decrease hospitalization, suffering, and suicide is the use of long-acting injectable medication. Long-acting injectables are antipsychotics that release the medication slowly over the course of weeks to months; the frequency depends on your client and the specific agent (See following table).

In order to ensure that your client is not allergic to the medication, that it does not cause intolerable side effects, and that it is effective, a week or more of oral medication is *always* given prior to the first injection. Once you give a long-acting injection, you cannot take it back, and it lasts weeks. Many clients find that they experience less abnormal movements on injectable medication than they did on the same medication taken in pill form. This may occur because injectable formulations are associated with consistent blood levels in contrast to fluctuating levels with oral medication.

Most long-acting injectables require an "overlap"—that is, a time during which the client continues to take their oral medication after receiving the first injection. The two exceptions to this rule are the monthly, long-acting form of paliperidone (marketed as Invega Sustenna®) and the tri-monthly, long-acting form of paliperidone (marketed as Trinza®). That is because paliperidone uses a different release strategy in the injectable form, which is a distinct advantage for clients who hate taking pills. However, clients will still need to take the oral form of paliperidone (Invega) before receiving any long-acting injectable to assure its tolerability (including not being allergic). This is also true when your client misses their shot: They will need to take oral medication for a short while after they receive their next injection.

Long-Acting Injectables

Type	Active Ingredient	Brand Name	Frequency of Injection	Oral Overlap Needed?
Typical	Fluphenazine	Prolixin Decanoate®	2 weeks	Several days, then decrease in half several more, then stop
Typical	Haloperidol	Haldol Decanoate®	4 weeks, but varies	1 week, then half dose for 1 week more
Atypical	Aripiprazole	Abilify Maintena®	4 weeks	2 weeks of full dose, then stop
Atypical	Aripiprazole	Aristada®	4-6 weeks	3 weeks, then stop
Atypical	Paliperidone	Invega Sustenna	4 weeks	No overlap needed
Atypical	Paliperidone	Invega Trinza®	3 months	No overlap needed
Atypical	Risperidone	Risperdal Consta	2 weeks	3 weeks, then stop
Atypical	Olanzapine	Zyprexa Relprevv®	2-4 weeks; Must be observed for 3 hours after each injection	No overlap

The typical antipsychotics that come in long-acting formulations are Haldol (haloperidol) and Prolixin (fluphenazine), which are used for the treatment of schizophrenia. Remember, these medications work for psychosis but do not provide mood stabilization or augment treatment for depression.

The atypical agents that come in long-acting form are Abilify Maintena and Aristada (both aripiprazole), Risperdal Consta (risperidone), Invega Sustenna and Trinza (both paliperidone), and Zyprexa Relprevv (olanzapine). The injectable form of olanzapine requires injections anywhere from every two to four weeks, but it can only be used by specifically approved clinics that have procedures in place to observe your client for three hours after every injection and have the capacity to provide emergency transport to a hospital in case of delirium or coma. As you can imagine, long-acting olanzapine is not commonly used for this very important reason. Consta requires an injection every two weeks. For some clients that is not a deterrent, as they've been on risperidone with good results, have not experienced adverse effects, want to continue that medication, and don't seem to mind the schedule.

Case Example

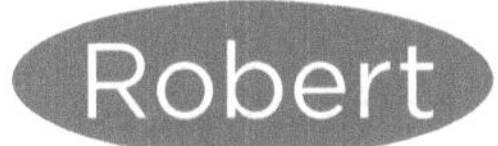

Robert, who was 46 years old when he came to see me, would start medication for his bipolar disorder with good intentions. But life would get in the way, and he wasn't really sure he needed the medication anyway, so he would start missing doses, become manic, and then completely stop the medication—causing him to lose his job and house, and prompting him to relapse on alcohol and methamphetamine to combat the ensuing depressive episode.

When I met Robert, he'd been repeating this pattern for about 20 years. After a short period of taking oral Invega (paliperidone), he started the long-acting injectable form (Sustenna). We set it up so he could easily come to the clinic first thing in the morning for his injection, usually seeing the same health assistant, and then get to his construction job.

When I recently switched him to Trinza, he commented that he had not experienced any manic episodes now for about a year and a half. He had experienced devastating manic episodes and depression at least twice a year for as long as he could remember. He shook his head in amazement that he could be this well. And when he learned his new long-acting injectable lasted three months, he smiled and said, "That's it? It's really this easy?"

> ## *Alert Your Client*
>
> The atypical agents that come in a long-acting formulation have different brand names than the same medication in pill form, even when made by the same drug company. For example, paliperidone is called Invega in pill form, Invega Sustenna in its monthly injectable formulation, and Invega Trinza in the three-month injectable formulation. It's all the same medication. Reassure your client if they are confused.

I frequently will give clients a trial of oral Invega (paliperidone), which is a similar molecule to risperidone, to see if they respond to that medication without adverse effects. After that oral pill trial, I change to the monthly injectable (Sustenna), which is given every four weeks. If they do well after four Sustenna injections, I can then change to Trinza, which requires a shot only every three months.

For clients who experience sedation on long-acting paliperidone, switching to long-acting aripiprazole can help. Long-acting Maintena or Aristada—both of which are aripiprazole, like oral Abilify—are also the injectables with the lowest risk of weight gain and increased blood glucose and lipids. Maintena must be given in the deltoid (arm) to get the full intended dose of the medication. If your client does well on Maintena but starts to experience symptoms during the last week before their next injection (e.g., hearing voices or feeling more depressed, hypomanic, or irritable), they may do better on longer-lasting Aristada, which can be given monthly in this situation but for other clients may last up to six weeks.

Why Long-Acting Injectables Matter

Clients who are on long-acting injectables spend significantly less days hospitalized—whether it be for psychiatric care, substance use disorder treatment, or some other cause. This translates into significantly less trauma and suffering for clients. They participate in outpatient treatment more frequently, and even with increased outpatient visits and the cost of injectable medication, their medical care costs are $10,000 less per year than clients on the oral form of the same medications (Lafeuille et al., 2014; Lefebvre et al., 2017). This finding is true for individuals with Medicaid, veterans, and those with co-occurring substance use and schizophrenia. Although long-acting injectable medications used to be considered a last-ditch effort for clients who were non-adherent with medication, they are actually more effective agents than oral medication and should be offered to clients regardless of their motivation to take medication. Perhaps this is part of the secret behind Europe's higher-recovery rates for schizophrenia than those in the United States: They are better at using long-acting injectables.

The tricky part is helping your client develop the willingness to even consider an injectable form of medication. When given the offer of a shot, most clients will quickly say, "No thanks." So how can you help clients take advantage of this

Case Example

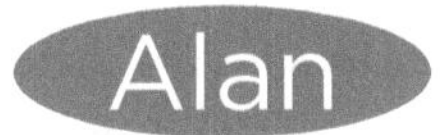

Alan, a 33-year-old man with schizophrenia and bipolar disorder, came to me just out of prison on oral Risperal (risperidone) and Klonopin (clonazepam). He was still having daily auditory hallucinations and significant paranoia, but he felt ambivalent about staying on antipsychotic medication. He did, however, want to continue taking Klonopin. We came to an agreement that I would keep him on Klonopin for the management of akathisia as long as he took Risperdal at an increased dose. He agreed.

As I met with him every two weeks, his paranoia and hallucinations gradually decreased. However, he hated having to take pills every day. After several months, he agreed to try the long-acting form of risperidone, Consta. After he had been on a few rounds of the injectable medication, his parole officer called to express how happy he was that Alan was conversing with him and was much less irritable. Shortly after, though, Alan grew tired of getting a shot every two weeks, so after a trial of oral Invega (paliperidone), he started Sustenna, which works for four weeks. He was pleased with this schedule and kept coming in every four weeks, in part motivated by his need to refill Klonopin at the same time. He contacted his children's mothers and began making regular contact, and he eventually started providing care for them on weekends.

Alan was relieved that he did not feel so paranoid, but he did not like how tired the medication made him feel. He was sleeping all night and still needed to nap during the day to counteract the sedation. So I switched him over to oral Abilify, and when he tolerated that, onto the injectable form (Maintena). His energy improved, and he lost most of the weight he'd gained on Consta. After a few months on Maintena, he came in with tears of happiness. He'd hosted a birthday party for his eight-year-old son, who then hugged him and asked if he would please host his birthday party again next year.

Alan has continued to improve on Maintena every month. He now cares for all three of his kids on weekends, attends their events, and tells stories of their school progress with pride. He's been off parole for several years. He continues on his long-acting injectable and low dose of Klonopin for the prevention of akathisia (and has never in four years asked for a higher dose).

medication form that we know decreases hospitalization rates by half? In my own experience, I found myself having very little success, so I spent time thinking about occasions when my clients went through the experience of being injected with an antipsychotic. I realized the experience was often connected to trauma, such as being involuntarily hospitalized or restrained, which is associated with the feeling of being completely out of control. Clearly, it was important to disassociate getting a shot from those experiences.

Therefore, I now reframe getting a monthly shot as something that is normal and about convenience—and I experience considerably more success. For example, in the course of my discussion about the hassle of taking pills every day, I mention that many women on birth control who don't want to risk missing any pills now choose to receive that protection in the form of a shot every month or at even longer intervals. This normalizes the experience and tends to increase interest in the conversation. I tell my clients how they could have that same option for their medication if that's something they might be interested in. It's important to emphasize they are in complete control in determining whether it's something they'd like to consider. If clients are amenable to this option, work with them to decrease any hassles and make the process of getting the shot as easy as possible. For example, some pharmacies now administer these shots, as do clinics with walk-in hours.

Alert Your Client

Think about delusions as a bleeding wound. When you are actively bleeding, that is what you focus on. Period. Therefore, the delusion is the constant focus of attention in the absence of treatment.

With treatment, though, the bleeding stops, the subsequent scab no longer becomes a constant focus, and your clients can turn their attention to life again. With medication, the brain is able to begin focusing on life. However, when you directly ask your clients about the delusion, it's like picking the scab—and, of course, it starts bleeding again.

Ask Your Client

The best time to ask your client if they have been offered the option of a long-acting injectable is when they are feeling frustrated or overwhelmed with the hassle of taking pills. Emphasize that it is normal for it to be hard to take pills every day. "That's why women get an easier, more convenient, and really effective way to take hormones when they really don't want to get pregnant. They just get a shot once a month or so, and that's it." Casually mention it as an analogous option for them. "Hmm, there may be that form for your medication too, let me see."

Give them the information we know: that long-acting injectables dramatically decrease hospitalization—something most clients would prefer to avoid—and have less side effects than pills do. Give examples of other clients who may have experienced success on monthly shots. Use motivational interviewing techniques. And above all, don't push. Instead, be somewhat nonchalant about it. "It's totally up to you. I guess if you wanted to think about it, we could let your prescriber know you'd like to consider it. It certainly would be easier, I get that."

Remember to stress to clients that they are in complete control. It is always completely up to them if they want to continue the injectable medication or return to taking it in pill form. "It's completely up to you and is only for your convenience. I get that it's sometimes a pain to take pills every day. But it's up to you." You get the idea.

Measuring Change in Psychosis

What you measure is more likely to change. It's true with mood disorders, and it's also true with psychosis. Here are a few effective ways I've found to measure change in psychosis. First, it is important to observe changes in functioning, although to get the internal experience of psychosis you need to go beyond simply asking, "How is it?" or "How bad are the voices?" Asking these questions is a first step, but many clients with schizophrenia have difficulty putting their experience into words. A metaphor can be helpful. One client of mine would share how his voices were either on "the back burner" or "the front burner" to describe when his symptoms were better or worse, respectively. Using this descriptor, he was able to successfully tell me when his hallucinations were intensifying and when they resolved again. He internally measured the frequency, intensity, and pervasiveness of the hallucinations using this metaphor. Prior to that, he would describe the voices as "bad" or "okay" but with much less specificity.

Second, a simple Likert scale also works amazingly well to measure change. Using a blank piece of paper, draw a line with 0 on one end and 5 on the other, and add hashmarks if you'd like. Instruct your client that 0 reflects no voices (or whatever symptom you are measuring) and 5 reflects the worst the symptoms have ever been. Use their language to describe the symptom, and then ask them to mark where on the scale it is now. You will find clients who are unable to describe the intensity or frequency of their symptoms with words can rate their experience on this scale. It also helps clients access their creativity, tap into the memory of their personal experience, and problem solve what they need to do in order to help their symptoms decrease to a lower number. These strategies are unique to the client and powerful for decreasing the distress connected to psychosis. It also helps you measure change.

Measuring progress with delusions is a different matter. Delusions rarely completely disappear. Instead, they recede into the background. If you ask a client about their delusion—one that has disappeared into the background due to the success of treatment—it will likely jump to the forefront again. For example, if you directly ask a client, "How has it been lately with that stalker outside the library?" they are likely to respond with "Oh, he's still there." This response leads you to incorrectly believe that there has been no improvement.

Instead, measure the amount of time in your interview that the client spends on non-delusional content when it comes to their life experiences, complaints, and concerns. As the amount of time increases before the delusion comes up, you know your client is improving. Conversely, when delusions worsen, there will be little to no time spent on non-delusional content.

Talking about psychosis is an extremely vulnerable thing for clients to do. Think about how you interact with clients who have history of trauma. Use those same strategies, such as changing pacing and shifting eye contact as appropriate, to create a safe space for those with psychosis. And most importantly, ask about their experiences. Clients who have experienced psychosis are in tune with what therapists and prescribing providers are willing and able to hear. Much like clients with other traumatic experiences, these clients will not share with you their experience of denigrating hallucinations, the fear of intense paranoia, or the intense isolation and loneliness that accompanies psychosis—not to mention the traumatic experiences of assault, humiliation, and loss they experience in health care settings and with law enforcement—unless you ask and are willing to hear their stories. Suicide is a significant cause of death for clients with schizophrenia, so take the time to listen.

Additional Ways to Improve Outcomes

Time is of the essence when it comes to helping clients with schizophrenia and other forms of psychosis stay stable and prevent decompensation. One effective strategy is to work with your clients to identify their earliest signs of "roughening" stability. It could involve not sleeping well, feeling alienated and alone, or other experiences that are not directly psychotic but have been a prelude to worsening psychosis in the past. Increased stressors, loss, and physical illness can precipitate these early warning signs.

Talk with your client about taking a PRN dose of their antipsychotic medication in these situations. Your support and assistance are invaluable in recognizing these "when I need it" times. Too often, even when clients have a PRN medication on hand, they don't recognize the early warning signs and fail to use it. Once the actual psychosis emerges, there is a narrow window of opportunity to use the PRN. If clients miss this window, they'll often lose insight into their need for medication, or they will develop delusions or auditory hallucinations telling them to stop medication. Adherence to medication is more highly correlated with your client's ability to recognize their own personal symptoms than their belief they have any mental illness.

The most effective strategy for helping clients stay on their antipsychotic medication is well-known: Reward them. Studies conducted in Europe have repeatedly demonstrated that providing clients with positive reinforcement increases medication adherence, even when it's a hassle to get to the pharmacy, in spite of annoying side effects, and regardless of whether they believe they need the medication (Noordraven, 2017, 2018). Rewards work.

Unfortunately, there is a bias against this evidence-based approach in the U.S. that stems from the fear that it is coercive to clients and deprives them of free choice. I don't know about you, but when I work—which can be stressful at times and causes me to feel tired, yet I continue to do it—I am indeed motivated by a dependable paycheck. I'm not convinced our clients with schizophrenia are any different. Have conversations with your client about how they can build in rewards, which might include talking with their protective payee together to see how they can get a special payment (or a movie ticket or bus pass) when they make it to the clinic and get their long-acting injection. Are there other people in your client's life who might be happy to send a monthly gift card in the same way? Most of us set up motivational and reward systems in our lives to keep doing what we need to, even when it's a hassle or unpleasant. Help your client develop a similar system to support their ongoing stability and health.

Vulnerable Populations

Pregnant Women

Antipsychotics are the mainstay of treatment for schizophrenia and one of the key medications in bipolar disorders. Traditionally, when treating psychosis in pregnant women, both typical and atypical antipsychotics have been used. However, in 2011 the FDA added a warning that certain antipsychotics can cause temporary abnormal movements, like dystonia, in newborns. These medications include all the typical antipsychotics and Risperdal (risperidone). In addition, the treatment of dystonia with Cogentin (benztropine) can have adverse effects on the developing baby, so all these medications should be avoided. The use of other atypical agents during pregnancy is not associated with birth defects (Huybrechts et al., 2016).

With these exceptions, the best antipsychotic medication is generally that which successfully treated the mother's illness prior to pregnancy. Be sure that your client's psychiatric prescriber and women's health care provider talk with each other. Your client may need your help in figuring out how to make that happen. Overall, the benefits that come from ensuring your client stays euthymic, stable, and nonpsychotic far outweigh the risks of most medications during pregnancy.

Youth

The use of antipsychotics in individuals under the age of 25 has significantly increased over the past decade. However, youth are extremely vulnerable to akathisia, weight gain, and metabolic adversity. For first-episode psychosis, atypical agents are first-line treatment because they build up the brain-derived neurotropic factor (BDNF) necessary for new neural connections to develop, which is crucial for recovery from a first episode of psychosis. Typical antipsychotics do not do this.

First-episode psychosis does not always proceed to schizophrenia, and one randomized controlled study found that adding omega-3 fatty acids for several months after a first episode of psychosis significantly decreased the rate at which individuals developed schizophrenia (Pawełczyk et al., 2016). Unfortunately, this result has not been replicated in subsequent studies. A low dose of an atypical antipsychotic, preferably one with a low incidence of weight gain, combined with wrap-around services promoting social reengagement, education, and occupational development is the treatment of choice.

For bipolar disorders, Risperdal, Abilify (aripiprazole), and Saphris (asenapine) are top-tier medications for the treatment of acute mania, whereas Latuda (lurasidone) is top-tier for the treatment of acute depression. Abilify is the medication of choice for maintenance of both these symptoms. Clearly, it's not helpful to switch a client with bipolar disorder around from agent to agent depending on their mood. These are just the first choices when thinking about both efficacy and safety.

Older Adults

Older adults are more vulnerable to developing tardive dyskinesia on antipsychotic medication, and as many as ten percent develop this movement disorder per year. The older typical antipsychotics, such as Haldol, are more likely than the atypical agents to trigger the development of this syndrome. The typicals are also more likely to cause dystonia, which requires Cogentin to treat that side effect. Unfortunately, Cogentin itself causes a variety of adverse effects in older adults, notably constipation, memory problems, and cognitive confusion. For these reasons, typical antipsychotics are not recommended for older adults.

There are additional risks to using atypical agents for older clients with dementia, including stroke and death. Therefore, these medications are not recommended as the initial treatment of choice for dementia-related agitation. Rather, the most effective, first-line treatment for agitation in dementia is a full evaluation of the psychosocial and living situation, followed by identifying and altering any sources of frustration.

When antipsychotics are absolutely necessary, the atypicals are generally preferred due to their decreased risk of dystonia and the need for Cogentin, which worsens dementia. The antipsychotic with the least risk of causing dystonia is Seroquel (quetiapine). Current guidelines suggest using atypical agents only when dementia-related agitation or psychosis is severe, potentially endangers the client or others, or causes the client significant distress (Bjerre et al., 2018). These agents should not be used long-term—that is, over four weeks—if they are not effective. Even if they are effective, they should be tapered down within four months to see if the client still needs the medication. Schizophrenia tends to attenuate in older adults, so your client may need less medication than before. Decreasing the dose decreases the adverse effects.

Autism Spectrum Disorders

Antipsychotics can be effective at reducing the agitation, self-injury, and aggression seen in youth with autism spectrum disorders (Wink et al., 2017). However, these clients are very sensitive to dystonia and akathisia, so they generally need lower doses of medications that are least likely to cause movement disorders, such as Seroquel. Unfortunately, these clients are also highly vulnerable to the weight gain associated with atypical agents. If your client is gaining weight, advocate for them with their provider to see about a medication that has a lower incidence of weight gain, or if it would be beneficial to add metformin or consider other alternatives. At times, though, the benefit of improved functioning outweighs the metabolic risks.

Co-occurring Substance Use Disorders

A common misconception is that medication should be stopped if a client is using substances. This is not true for most prescription psychiatric medications, and it's definitely not true of antipsychotics. It is also a myth that antipsychotic medications won't work if your client is using substances. Antipsychotics will treat psychosis even if it is caused or worsened by substance use. Therefore, while it is important to differentiate substance-induced psychosis from other forms of psychosis for the purpose of treatment planning, from a purely medicinal perspective, it is not critical.

Obviously, it is a good idea for a client with psychosis to abstain from using methamphetamines, as it makes it more challenging to treat underlying psychotic symptoms. But medications do still work in these circumstances. It is important for professionals to understand the efficacy of antipsychotic medication when working with individuals who have a co-occurring substance use disorder, as it otherwise generates an apathy that leaves these clients undertreated.

Ask Your Client

Ask your client directly, "Do you take your medication when you use drugs or alcohol?" Many clients stop taking their medication when they engage in substance use because they are afraid of dangerous interactions. For antipsychotics, there are no such interactions, with the possible exception of Geodon (ziprasidone), which should not be prescribed or taken with methadone. So ask. I tell my clients that their brain becomes more vulnerable when they use alcohol and drugs, so that is a time when their brain needs their medication more than ever. Encourage them to check with their prescriber as well. Then, encourage them to keep taking their antipsychotic medication even—and especially—when they are using substances.

At the same time, there are some concerns for the misuse of antipsychotic medication when clients have an active substance abuse disorder. In particular, clients will often misuse Seroquel by using it to help them "come down" from the high of other drugs and sleep. Clients usually desire lower dosages (25-100 mg tablets) for this purpose, so when I have this concern, I tend not to prescribe Seroquel in such low doses, or I choose a different medication.

Conclusion

In summary, antipsychotic medications effectively treat more than psychosis and can make a remarkable difference in your clients' lives. However, for most clients with schizophrenia and bipolar disorders, taking medication is a daunting, lifelong commitment. Your role is critical in helping clients integrate that reality into their sense of self in such a manner that promotes self-compassion and acceptance and minimizes shame. In addition, since these agents are associated with significant inconveniences and can carry significant side effects, make sure to ask questions and reassure your client that alternatives exist, such as different medications or the use of a long-acting injectable for convenience. Stopping their medication is not the only answer. Help them connect to and make changes with their provider that can make the process of taking medication as little of a hassle as possible. Above all, focus on helping your client recover, which involves creating a meaningful life that brings them satisfaction and joy, as well as accepting the limitations and necessities of their illness (which includes taking medication).

Chapter 5

Treatment of Anxiety Disorders

Anxiety disorders are the most common psychiatric condition, as studies estimate that anywhere between 17 and 30 percent of the population is affected by this condition at some point in their life (Bandelow & Michaelis, 2015; Somers et al., 2006). There are many faces of anxiety, ranging from panic attacks and difficulty leaving the house to jitteriness and constant worry. The onset of certain anxiety disorders (separation anxiety disorder, social anxiety disorder, and specific phobias) occurs most frequently in childhood and early adolescence, whereas other types of anxiety (OCD, panic disorder, and generalized anxiety disorder) are most likely to develop in early adulthood (Lijster et al., 2017).

Anxiety can be mildly annoying or severely disabling, and it is highly comorbid with other mental disorders, particularly major depressive disorder. In fact, it is much more difficult to fully treat major depressive disorder when there is a comorbid, untreated anxiety disorder. In addition, clients with co-occurring anxiety and mood disorders are at an increased risk of suicidality compared to those with a single mood disorder (Sareen et al., 2005).

The most effective treatment for anxiety is psychotherapy, particularly CBT, with medication playing an important, supporting role. For severe anxiety disorders, and particularly with panic disorder, medication may be critical. In this chapter, I will review the medications that can benefit your client and how they work. I'll also provide a detailed review regarding the advantages and dangers of benzodiazepines, which are the most commonly prescribed agent for anxiety. I'll suggest specific strategies you can use when you have concerns about the benzodiazepines your clients are taking and outline an approach to increase their motivation to talk with their prescriber and try alternatives. In addition, I'll review other classes of agents, both prescription and supplemental, that are highly effective at treating anxiety, while highlighting the important role of psychotherapy.

Neurobiology of Anxiety

While we do not know exactly what causes anxiety disorders, we do know the neurotransmitters involved and what agents are helpful. For example, serotonin is heavily involved in anxiety, as evidenced by the fact that SSRIs, which work on only serotonin, are highly effective in treating anxiety. Similarly, we know anxiety is also connected to an imbalance in two other neurotransmitters: GABA (the calming neurotransmitter) and glutamate (the excitatory neurotransmitter). GABA and glutamate are inversely related in that when GABA goes up, glutamate goes down, resulting in a sense of calmness and relaxation. In contrast, when glutamate goes up, GABA goes down, resulting in more energy, anxiety, or agitation. Normally, these neurotransmitters are balanced, but a number of things can dysregulate this balance, particularly the experience of trauma.

While PTSD is no longer considered an anxiety disorder in the latest edition of the *Diagnostic and Statistical Manual of Mental Disorders* (APA, 2013), individuals with a trauma history often present with high anxiety. This is because, in addition to disrupting the balance between GABA and glutamate, trauma causes long-term changes in the hypothalamic-pituitary-adrenal system that governs the amount of cortisol released in the body. In particular, chronic trauma results in prolonged elevations of cortisol, which adversely affects both the body and brain. When the adrenal gland eventually becomes exhausted with this long-term, excess production of cortisol, adrenal insufficiency occurs, which results in more infections, illnesses, and vulnerability to anxiety. Indeed, the groundbreaking Adverse Childhood Experiences (ACEs) Study found that children exposed to early childhood adversity experience a cascade of brain and body changes associated with impaired development, risky health behaviors, increased risk of developing a chronic disease, and earlier death (Felitti et al., 1998).

While the most effective treatments for anxiety focus primarily on serotonin and GABA, the actual neural mechanisms contributing to anxiety are thought to be more connected to the fight-or-flight response. In particular, specific neuroanatomical regions in the amygdala or hypothalamus may be easily overactivated in clients with anxiety disorders, making them more vulnerable to unprovoked panic when exposed to either internal or environmental stimuli. Therefore, it is likely that the combination of an underlying genetic predisposition combined with certain vulnerability factors, such as adversity or stress, precipitates the onset of anxiety disorders.

Getting the Diagnosis Right

Anxiety is one of those common concerns that tells you virtually nothing about what is going on. Clients use "bad anxiety" to describe many experiences, and those experiences may have a range of etiologies. When your client reports feeling "anxious," they may be talking about their experience of frequent worry, or they may be referring to panic attacks, depression, a sense of impending doom, or the restlessness of akathisia. All these conditions are commonly referred to as "anxiety." In addition, while these experiences may reflect an underlying anxiety disorder, they could also be caused by excessive caffeine intake, an overactive thyroid, low oxygen levels (e.g., from chronic obstructive pulmonary disease or sleep apnea), or medication side effects, just to name a few causes. Don't assume you know exactly what your client means by "anxiety" or that they have an anxiety disorder at all. Encourage your clients to visit a primary care provider to rule out alternative explanations for their experience.

Ask Your Client

Ask your client these key questions in distinguishing the source of their anxiety:

1. "Would you say you feel anxiety more in your brain or your body? For example, do you find yourself worrying or ruminating a lot, or do you have more physical symptoms, like hyperventilating, restless legs, or racing heart?"

2. "Is the anxiety worse at certain times and better at other times? Or is it pretty much constant?"

3. "How is it when you are home in familiar surroundings? How about when you think about going out?"

4. "Describe your last panic attack. What did you notice first? Then what happened? How long did it last? What did you do to manage it?"

5. "Has anything changed? New medication, new sleep arrangements, new stressors?"

Benzodiazepines

Benzodiazepines are the most frequently prescribed type of medication for anxiety disorders. Common benzodiazepines include Ativan (lorazepam), Klonopin (clonazepam), Valium® (diazepam), and Xanax® (alprazolam). These medications work by increasing GABA and decreasing glutamate. Benzodiazepines work on the $GABA_A$ receptor site on the post-synaptic neuron. They are rapidly absorbed into the blood and brain, with Xanax being the most rapid. Rapid onset of action is what makes a substance more addictive, which is why Xanax tends to be more addictive than other benzodiazepines, although all have addictive potential. Benzodiazepines are effective, but they also have the significant potential for harm. The adverse effects fall into three categories: **(1)** psychological effects, **(2)** dangerous drug interactions, and **(3)** physical effects.

Adverse Effects of Benzodiazepines

First, there are the adverse psychological effects to consider. There is a syndrome that occurs with the long-term use of benzodiazepines at higher doses that is characterized by difficulty making decisions, feeling more powerless and helpless, avoidance of social responsibilities, and an increased focus on the medication as the source of one's competence. This results in frequent requests for a higher dose, use of the medication to eliminate difficult feelings, and a reduction in functioning in the world. Clients feel it is increasingly critical to use benzodiazepines to stave off anxiety, and the dose isn't enough. Their anxiety symptoms become poorly controlled, in spite of higher doses of medication.

Some of your clients on benzodiazepines may have experienced this syndrome when their prescriber decides to stop prescribing these medications. The pattern goes something like this: The prescriber becomes worried or frustrated about the client's benzodiazepine usage and decides to stop prescribing, perhaps giving a short-term prescription of two weeks to taper off. As you know, what most frequently happens is that your client finds a different prescriber. The whole experience then fuels the client's fear to talk about discontinuing the medication in the future.

The second concern regarding benzodiazepines is their potential for serious harm or death when used in combination with other central nervous system depressants. Opiates and alcohol are of particular concern, as both agents cause respiratory depression and increase the potential for lethality. Using multiple central nervous system depressants can cause your client to stop breathing at night and die. The huge majority of deaths from opiate overdose result from taking multiple agents, with benzodiazepines being the most frequently used agent in this lethal combination. **At the risk of oversimplification, remember the following rule of thumb: Opiates + Benzodiazepines = Death.** Therefore, benzodiazepines should not be prescribed for clients who engage in problematic alcohol or opiate use, or even those who engage in regular, nonproblematic use. Be sure to alert the prescriber if your client is given a prescription for a benzodiazepine and they regularly use opiates or drink alcohol.

The third issue to consider is that benzodiazepines can also have other physical adverse effects. They often cause memory difficulties, both in terms of learning new information and remembering old information. Even if a client does not have cognitive impairment to begin with, benzodiazepines can worsen memory. "I keep losing things" is a common complaint that clients may make without recognizing it as an adverse effect of the medication. Clients may also have a more difficult time learning new information in a class or on the job. This effect holds true for both short- and long-term use, although the problem occurs most often with high dosing and long-term use.

Benzodiazepines also increase the risk of Alzheimer's disease, with the risk increasing with the dose and length of time taken. This is one reason why benzodiazepines are on the Beers list, a well-recognized American Geriatrics Society list of medications to be avoided in older adults (American Geriatrics Society Beers Criteria Update Expert Panel, 2019). However, you can imagine benzodiazepines are not helpful for clients of any age who have dementia and milder neurocognitive problems.

In addition, benzodiazepines increase fall risk. Again, your client may not connect their falling with the medication. Unfortunately, older, and often frail, women receive more prescriptions for benzodiazepines than any other population in America. Don't underestimate the danger of falling for your client. Head injuries and broken hips are catalysts for a cascade of ill effects.

Finally, benzodiazepines cause psychomotor impairment. Although clients may acclimate to the sedating effect of these agents, the underlying psychomotor impairment does not subside. This means that while your client may feel alert while

Case Example

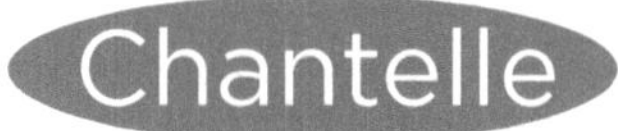

Chantelle, a 27-year-old woman, was in tears when she spoke with me. A new client of mine, she had just been—in her words—"kicked out" of care by her prescriber, who'd given her a two-week prescription of Xanax (alprazolam) with one refill. The prescriber had instructed her to taper off the medication herself and told her that it would be the last prescription she would get.

I asked Chantelle about her history of taking Xanax, and she reported it was first given to her six years ago for the treatment of infrequent panic attacks. She was initially prescribed 0.5 mg twice a day, but the symptoms returned and her dose was increased, eventually up to 2 mg three times a day. This higher dosage worked for a while, but the anxiety, which had now become more pervasive, and panic attacks would return. She eventually found it hard to go to work and switched to a part-time job close to her apartment.

She started supplementing her prescriptions with whatever she could find from her sister's medicine cabinet. "It works, but it's just not enough." Her medical bills were piling up, as she'd been to the emergency room on various occasions for panic attacks, where she was frequently given immediate relief with Ativan (lorazepam). She didn't know what to do. She was likely getting evicted at the end of the month, with no money for rent. "The only thing that works is the Xanax. I can't live without it."

driving to work, their psychomotor ability to drive is still impaired. Your client needs to know they can be arrested for driving under the influence from benzodiazepines, even when they don't feel sleepy.

When to Avoid Benzodiazepines: Clients and Conditions to Consider

Given their long list of adverse effects, it helps to think of benzodiazepines as a double-edged sword with potential for great help and great harm. The trick is how to use these agents to get the benefit without the harm. The first step is knowing which clients are good candidates and for what conditions these medications are most helpful. And conversely, you should know when the dangers outweigh the potential benefits.

Topping the list of clients for whom the potential danger outweighs benefit are clients with a history of benzodiazepine addiction or misuse. The brain never forgets benzodiazepines. If your client struggled with benzodiazepines 20 years ago, taking one now is likely to trigger cravings and misuse. Slightly lower down the list is any client who is currently struggling with the misuse of substances other than benzodiazepines, such as alcohol. These clients can tolerate benzodiazepines after getting clean and sober. Once they have been sober for at least one year, then benzodiazepines may be an option—provided their anxiety disorder is life-impairing (e.g., they are unable to work) and other medications and CBT have not helped. In these cases, benzodiazepines may actually lower the client's risk of relapsing on alcohol and or substances (Posternak & Mueller, 2001).

The dangers of benzodiazepines also outweigh the benefits for clients with PTSD. Although these clients are often prescribed benzodiazepines to counteract PTSD-associated anxiety and insomnia, the use of benzodiazepines can exacerbate their symptoms and prolong the healing process because they disrupt memory (re)consolidation. Similarly, clients who have just been exposed to a recent traumatic experience should not take benzodiazepines, as they interfere with the brain's ability to process the acute exposure and heal during sleep. Taking a benzodiazepine blocks this natural process and increases the risk of PTSD.

Other groups of clients for whom the dangers likely outweigh the benefits are older adults, clients on methadone or other opiates (respiratory depression and death), and those with sleep apnea (also respiratory depression). It is also important to consider whether clients have family members with a current or past addiction to benzodiazepines, as these clients are at higher risk of falling into misuse and addiction themselves. Caution should also be taken with youth and women who are pregnant (see Vulnerable Populations section).

In addition, there are several groups of clients who do not typically benefit from benzodiazepines. For example, clients with a traumatic brain injury, autism spectrum disorders, or intellectual disabilities tend to respond paradoxically to these medications, meaning that it has an agitating effect instead of a calming effect. It can also cause them to engage in impulsive, disinhibited behaviors, such as disrobing in public settings, or engaging in uncharacteristic gambling, sexual, or aggressive

Case Example

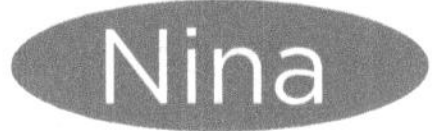

Nina was a 54-year-old woman with a lifelong phobia of needles. Although she had navigated life without it causing her much distress, she was now nearing kidney failure. She was refusing to go to dialysis, and her family was beside themselves. "Every time I even think about going—and I'm supposed to go twice a week—I just freeze. I can't do it."

Nina had no history of alcohol or drug problems, and although she had a history of depressive episodes, she was not currently depressed. We talked about options, including an SSRI, but decided to try a low dose of Xanax (alprazolam). She took 0.25 mg in the mornings she was scheduled for dialysis. She returned smiling and said, "I can do it!"

She found that this low dose allowed her to tolerate the dialysis procedure ("It's not great, but it works"). She didn't experience any sedation later in the day and otherwise reported feeling "fine."

behaviors. Clients with serious mental illnesses have also historically been over-prescribed benzodiazepines for sleep and agitation.

Even with all these potential problems, it is important to remember there is a "good edge" to the sword of benzodiazepines. These are highly effective agents, and many clients do very well on them, even when taking them for years. They work extremely well for the short-term treatment of anxiety, specific phobias, grief (e.g., following the expected death of a loved one, not sudden trauma), and insomnia. Over the long term, they are also effective in the treatment of panic disorder and the akathisia associated with antipsychotic medications. Many clients take them without any problem.

Another factor that distinguishes the good edge of benzodiazepines from the dangers is the dose. The table below provides a useful reference for the dosing ranges associated with the likely safe usage of benzodiazepines, as well as those of possible concern. This is simply a guideline, though, so you should continue to watch your clients for adverse effects and assess for efficacy, and be mindful of benzodiazepine usage that is likely connected to problems. Your individual client's circumstances may mean they need a lower dose of the medication to be safe, or a higher dose for it to be effective.

Dosing of Benzodiazepines

Name	Probably Safe	Watch and Assess	Problems Likely
Ativan (lorazepam)	Under 6 mg	6-10 mg	Over 10 mg
Klonopin (clonazepam)	Under 1.5 mg	1.5-3 mg	Over 3 mg
Valium (diazepam)	Under 20 mg	20-40 mg	Over 40 mg
Xanax (alprazolam)	Under 3 mg	3-5 mg	Over 5 mg

If the dosing is in the "probably safe" column, the medication is working well, and your client doesn't exhibit any of the previous concerns, then you probably don't need to worry about them. These clients tend to continue to do well on the medication and are unlikely to develop a tolerance or ask for increases in dosage. Clients in the "watch and assess" column are more likely to request increased doses in the medication that may or may not be warranted. Clients in the "problems likely" column, who are taking the highest dose, frequently have the psychological syndrome described earlier characterized by feeling powerless and overwhelmed by life—and yet they still feel like their medication is not working. These are the clients that need your help.

When your client is in this "problems likely" zone, carefully assess for adverse impacts and determine if their anxiety disorder is well-treated. Most likely it is not, but your client has probably given up hope it can be better and deeply fears losing the little help they do get from their benzodiazepine. Suggest to these clients that they deserve better (and safer!) treatment, more joy, and less pain in life. And here's how to support them to get there: Motivate them to talk to their prescriber and share their willingness to consider the possibility of discontinuing benzodiazepines in lieu of other treatment options. You can also communicate with their prescriber (with their permission) about your client's observed problems and continued anxiety.

Alert Your Client

Benzodiazepines cannot be "just stopped" without potentially dangerous effects. Alcohol and benzodiazepines are two substances that can be medically dangerous to stop using without tapering down or using a substitute medication to prevent seizures and other complications.

Discontinuing Benzodiazepines

Discontinuing benzodiazepines can be a good choice when the dangers outweigh the benefits. But many clients become highly attached to this medication and may have had stressful experiences in the past with a prescriber cutting them off. You play an important role in this process by (1) successfully motivating your client to talk with their prescriber about different treatment options, (2) clarifying and confirming the exact anxiety disorder diagnosis, (3) making any needed adjustments to your therapy plan to target their anxiety, and (4) supporting them during a taper and trial of new medication. In doing so, you provide your client with an opportunity to receive better treatment that will improve their functioning and well-being.

First, pay attention to the association between the use of benzodiazepines and whatever adverse effects your client is experiencing. For example, if your client complains about memory problems and falls, help them understand that these problems are a possible side effect of the medication. Clients can be relieved to learn this if they are worried they are developing dementia. Second, listen for concerns that the medication is "not enough" or that clients "need just one more pill" to treat their condition, as this indicates that not only are they experiencing adverse effects, but their anxiety disorder is also not being treated successfully. Third, pay attention to the hassles they experience when it comes to their benzodiazepine usage—from their prescriber refusing to write a new prescription, to the pharmacy denying a refill request because it is "too soon," to insurance coverage issues. Help your client recognize this trifecta: adverse effects, inadequately treated anxiety, and hassles.

In addition, there is one more critical element to support your client in considering alternative forms of treatment. Your client needs to know that you deeply understand how awful it is for them to experience anxiety. So get into the details regarding their experience. Until your client is absolutely sure that you fully understand the breadth and depth of their anxiety, you will be unable to help them consider better treatment options and they will be unwilling to talk with their prescriber about better (and maybe safer) types of medication.

Ask Your Client

Ask your client about their unique "fingerprint" of anxiety. It is not enough to know they have panic attacks. Find out what the experience is like for them. What happened that time they had a panic attack in their son's classroom? What did it feel like? What were they thinking about themselves, or about their ability as a parent? What was it like when they were unable to attend their son's parent-teacher conference because of social anxiety? How often does anxiety trigger that shame experience? What were their thoughts and feelings connected to these experiences? What is it like to worry about having a panic attack? How many hours a day does this consume?

Of course, the goal is to decrease your client's suffering and improve their health, not just to get rid of benzodiazepines. Reframing the goal in this manner changes everything. It's no longer about taking away benzodiazepines; it's about helping your client feel better. It's very powerful to watch your client go from feeling powerless to believing they deserve and have the right to expect better treatment—and that better care includes therapy as well as medication.

In order to develop a plan to better treat your client, it is critical to conduct a thorough differential diagnostic assessment. Does the client also have a mood disorder? Psychosis? Insomnia? Are there multiple anxiety disorders? Do they have an underlying trauma history? Taking time to excavate your client's unique history, symptom presentation, and diagnostic profile is immensely helpful in improving their treatment because there are many alternative medications that are equally as effective as benzodiazepines in treating anxiety. The specific type of anxiety disorder, as well as individual health issues and co-occurring disorders, can all determine which agents are best.

Therefore, communicate the results of your diagnostic assessment with the prescriber, outline your revised therapy plan, and—very importantly—list the concerns about benzodiazepines you identified with your client. Tell them your client is *interested in considering medication options and is open to tapering off benzodiazepines.* Share your plan to meet regularly with your mutual client during this time, given that regularly addressing progress (and challenges) in each therapy session improves the likelihood your client will be successful in tapering off benzodiazepines.

While discontinuing benzodiazepines may or may not be what the prescriber recommends, it is only part of the overall plan to provide that "better care." Gradually stopping benzodiazepines is a means to an end, but it is not the goal. What exactly is the goal? Less anxiety, of course. But what exactly does that look like for clients? Have them describe how they picture their life without anxiety. The more specific and detailed they can be, the better. Communicate that identified goal with the prescriber as well.

The Taper

When your client finally begins the discontinuation process, there are several medications that can decrease discomfort and increase the likelihood of a successful taper. Some of these agents include Tegretol (carbamazepine), Depakote (valproate), and trazodone (Guaiana & Barbui, 2016). Many clients find that taking a low dose of one of these agents multiple times a day is helpful. Typically, clients will take 250 mg of Depakote, 100-200 mg of Tegretol, or 25 mg (or less) of trazodone in the morning and afternoon, with a larger dose at bedtime. Although it will not feel like their usual experience of benzodiazepine, it will take the edge off of their anxiety.

It is very difficult to taper off short-acting benzodiazepines, particularly Xanax. Your client is likely to have uncomfortable, worsened anxiety between doses and abandon the plan. Clients who are on Xanax are usually changed over to a longer-acting agent, such as Klonopin or Ativan. However, Klonopin is extremely potent and can cause its own problems, as it is very easy for clients to end up in the higher-dosing range while seemingly on very little. For example, a client taking 1 mg of Klonopin is on the same amount of benzodiazepine as a client taking 4 mg of Ativan (see below). It is psychologically harder to taper off a medication such as Klonopin when on such a low milligram dose. Additionally, the drug is not readily available in low enough doses to taper down without having to break pills in half. A client tapering off a benzodiazepine will have great difficulty breaking pills in half. It usually doesn't happen.

In contrast, Ativan is a mid-length acting agent with a higher milligram equivalency, causing the medication to psychologically feel like more, and it comes in small enough doses that clients can taper down without having to break pills in half. A client taking 1 mg of Klonopin twice a day (the equivalent of 8 mg of Ativan) is likely to feel more confident when tapering down if they are switched to 6 mg of Ativan instead of 1.5 mg of Klonopin (both a drop of 25 percent).

Potency of Common Benzodiazepines

Name	Potency Equivalent	Length of action
Xanax (alprazolam)	0.5 mg	Very short 3-4 hours
Ativan (lorazepam)	1 mg	Mid-length 6 hours
Klonopin (clonazepam)	0.25 mg	Long 8 hours
Valium (diazepam)	5 mg	Very long (12+ hours)—dangerous with older adults

Tapering the dose gradually over a substantial period of time is the recommended strategy. For example, decreasing the dose by 25 percent every two weeks, or by 10 percent weekly. I find it challenging to manage weekly prescriptions, so I prefer to drop it by 25 percent every two weeks. This 25 percent decrease reflects the percentage of the current dose, not the original dose, so it creates a taper with a long, slow tail. This taper pattern is helpful to clients because while the largest decrease happens early in the taper, it is the last 1 mg of medication that is the most challenging, so it allows clients to go even slower toward the end.

Alternatively, some prescribers use a plan that involves dropping the dose by 25 percent for the first two weeks, then dropping it by 50 percent and holding that dose for a month, and then slowly tapering off thereafter (Ogbonna & Lembke, 2017). It is normal for the taper to take anywhere from three to six months. The specific taper pattern and length should be determined in accordance with your client's individual needs.

Never assume your client will be able to break a pill in half in this process. If the prescriber has written the prescription with instructions to break the pill in half, your client can take it to the pharmacy and request assistance with cutting them in half ahead of time. I see clients every two weeks during this process until they gain confidence the plan is actually working and can move to monthly visits.

In addition, when you meet with your client during this process, always assume they have used extra benzodiazepines over the taper prescribed. Never ask, "Did you take any extra medication?" because you will always get a resounding "no" and compromise your collaboration. Assume they are needing and using other benzodiazepines.

Ask Your Client

Instead of asking if your client supplemented their taper with extra benzodiazepines, ask them how they did so. It helps normalize the difficulty involved in the discontinuation process. "Cutting down on your benzodiazepine can be hard. Many times, people get triggered and find they need to take extra. How's that for you?" You can follow up by asking specific questions to determine what triggered their need to take the additional medication. "How often did you have that happen? What was going on then?" Oftentimes, the trigger involves a situation, person, or particular time of day. Help them distinguish if this trigger reflected rebound anxiety, their underlying anxiety disorder, or adverse effects from the taper.

Common experiences in tapering off benzodiazepines include fatigue, restlessness, agitation, insomnia, ringing ears, sweating, nausea, increased sensitivity to auditory or visual stimuli, and a sense of depersonalization. Many clients won't experience any of these symptoms, while for others it can cause extreme distress. If your client is struggling, encourage them to talk with their prescriber about alternative medication to assist with these symptoms—the goal is not suffering. In addition, reassure your client that these symptoms pose no medical danger.

Even with a gradual reduction in dose, there are four patterns of withdrawal that can occur: **(1)** a gradual, slow decrease in withdrawal severity, **(2)** an initial worsening in rebound anxiety followed by a decrease over time, **(3)** increasing severity as the taper progresses, and **(4)** no withdrawal at all. The last ten percent of the taper and the period immediately following complete discontinuation are frequently the worst in terms of rebound anxiety and withdrawal symptoms (Lader, 2014).

Don't forget to give kudos to your client each step of the way and reflect on their success. Talk about specifically what they notice is different. How do they see therapy and other parts of the treatment plan making a difference? Measure their anxiety so they can concretely see improvement each step of the way.

Treating Anxiety with Other Agents

For clients who still require medication for the treatment of their anxiety disorder, there are several alternatives that are equally as effective as benzodiazepines. These classes of medications include the antidepressants, anticonvulsants, antihypertensives, and antihistamines. BuSpar (buspirone), which is in its own class of medication, is another effective option. Some of these medications are more effective in targeting the psychomotor symptoms of anxiety (e.g., hyperventilation, rapid heart rate, sweaty palms, stomach "butterflies"), whereas others are more effective in addressing the cognitive worries and fears, such as those found in generalized anxiety disorder and social anxiety disorder.

Time Frame for Action in Treating Anxiety

Type of Agent	Action Time Frame
Antidepressants: SSRIs, SNRIs, Tricyclics	Take 1-2 months to work, after which they provide sustained relief (e.g., 24 hours/day)
Anticonvulsants	Provide immediate action; last for several hours
Antihistamines	Provide immediate action; last for several hours
Antihypertensives	Provde immediate actions; last for several hours
Atypical antipsychotics	Provide immediate action; last for hours but not recommended as first-line agents
BuSpar (buspirone)	Takes 1-2 months to work, after which it provides sustained relief (e.g., 24 hours/day)

Antidepressants for Anxiety

The SSRIs, SNRIs, and tricyclic antidepressants are all effective agents for treating anxiety disorders, including panic disorder (Bighelli et al., 2016). SSRIs are usually the first choice in terms of their efficacy and overall fewer adverse effects. However, many clients with anxiety disorders will say "I can't take them," likely referring to the experiences of akathisia they had from an SSRI started at the usual starting dose. Clients with anxiety disorders are exquisitely sensitive to akathisia and will quickly

Case Example

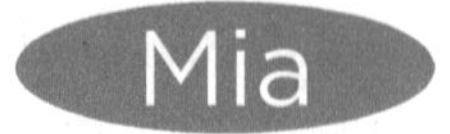

Mia, who was 31 years old, suffered with panic disorder and generalized anxiety disorder, which both interfered with her ability to work and function in her family. She had tried several different medications, including multiple SSRIs (which gave her intolerable "nerves"), Cymbalta (duloxetine—which left her feeling very sedated), and Effexor (venlafaxine—which also made her nervous). When she was tried on Ativan (lorazepam), it temporarily helped, but its efficacy soon wore off and she began to engage in problematic alcohol use as a means of coping with her anxiety. Although using alcohol helped slow down the anxiety, it made her angry and irritable, and her relationships with her partner and children suffered. She was reluctantly seeing a therapist, although she didn't believe it was helping. During this time, Mia was having daily panic attacks and would call my clinic multiple times a week asking for another pill.

Working with her therapist helped her to stop drinking, and the conflict at home improved, but her panic disorder continued to be problematic. We tried a different SSRI and added BuSpar (buspirone) for the generalized anxiety disorder, but without benefit. After she had been sober for several months, Mia agreed to a trial of a tricyclic antidepressant (25 mg of nortriptyline). After two weeks, Mia reported her panic attacks were gone. She was very surprised at the lack of anxiety and panic, and she reported she was sleeping better. The only side effect she had was constipation, so she began a regimen to assist with this, and I instructed her to return in two more weeks. Unfortunately, the constipation worsened during this time and she also developed urinary retention (difficulty urinating). Her primary care provider and I decided to stop the nortriptyline. These problems resolved, but her panic attacks returned. She tried other medications with only limited improvement and finally agreed to a more intensive trial of CBT.

She is now working again, with reductions in anxiety and panic, and she experiences less distress when panic attacks do occur.

throw away their medication if they feel jittery—because, of course, akathisia feels like worsened anxiety.

When SSRIs are used to treat anxiety, they need to be started at 10 to 25 percent of the usual starting dose to prevent akathisia and then titrated to an effective dose. Usually, treating anxiety requires higher doses than what works for depression. Reassure your client this is normal. Clients with anxiety disorders usually tolerate these higher SSRI doses well, provided it was originally started very low and then gradually titrated up.

If a client is having adverse effects or doesn't improve even in the higher dose range, trying a different agent is reasonable. Trying a second SSRI is equally as effective as trying an SNRI. Even if the second SSRI is in the same class of medication, the molecules are different enough that they vary in terms of side effects and effectiveness. One SSRI may not work, but the next may be highly effective.

Although tricyclic antidepressants are not well-known for their efficacy in treating anxiety, they are as effective as benzodiazepines. However, I have yet to convince my clients of this prior to a trial. The tricyclics have several advantages over other antidepressants, as they are less likely to cause akathisia, and most clients like their sedating effect, which helps with insomnia. Another advantage is that many clients have not been on these agents and are more willing to give them a try. The downside, of course, includes the usual tricyclic side effects, which are not minor. The risk of death on overdose tends to be less of a concern unless your client also has a mood disorder, but always ask about suicidality. Remember: Having a comorbid anxiety and mood disorder increases the risk of suicidality.

Other antidepressants, such as Cymbalta (duloxetine), Effexor (venlafaxine), Remeron (mirtazapine), and Wellbutrin (bupropion), work for the treatment of generalized anxiety, panic, and social anxiety disorder, although the data is not as strong as SSRIs. In contrast to SSRIs, which typically require higher doses than needed for depression, these agents can improve the anxiety disorder at usual doses, although the dose should be increased if there is no response. These agents also tend not to "poop out" like the SSRIs are known to do.

All antidepressants take time to work. For anxiety, outcomes continue to improve over three to six months after starting the medication. However, when clients are in acute distress, that can feel like an eternity. Combining a trial of an antidepressant with a more immediate-acting anxiolytic helps clients tolerate the wait. Once antidepressant medications do work, they provide sustained action and work 24 hours a day.

Anticonvulsants for Anxiety

Anticonvulsants have recently become more popular for treating anxiety, though evidence regarding their efficacy is not as strong. In addition to its utility when tapering off benzodiazepines, Depakote (valproate) can promote a mild anti-anxiety effect, which may be due to its sedative properties. Tegretol (carbamazepine) is not typically used for anxiety, other than preventing discomfort in tapering off benzodiazepines.

Gabapentin, on the other hand, albeit with limited data, is frequently prescribed for generalized anxiety—as well as the "cognitive" part of anxiety, regardless of diagnosis. Data indicates it is also effective in treating social anxiety disorder and in decreasing the anxiety and cravings related to discontinuation of alcohol (Ahmed et al., 2019; Mason, Quello, & Shadan, 2018). Gabapentin is sedating, but this effect wears off, so clients who can initially only tolerate 100 mg at night may be able to increase to a therapeutic dose, often taken three times daily, without increased sedation. It is usually prescribed to be taken multiple times a day, with a higher dose at bedtime. Gabapentin also works right away and lasts for several hours. The dosing is highly variable and can range anywhere from 100 mg a day to 3600 mg a day for the treatment of other conditions in primary care. It can be abused, as it increases the "high" experienced with opiates and thus has "street" value. Lyrica (pregabalin) is a medication similar to gabapentin that is approved for the treatment of social anxiety and generalized anxiety in Europe. However, it has not been approved in the U.S. and is also very expensive. That combination makes it unusual for clients to be prescribed Lyrica for anxiety.

Antihypertensives for Anxiety

Clonidine is a medication used to treat hypertension that is commonly prescribed for sleep and, more recently, anxiety. It works primarily through its fast-acting sedative effect, which for highly anxious clients can feel like a decrease in anxiety. It is most often combined with other agents to treat anxiety disorders. Alert your client that if they are taking more than 0.2 mg daily, they should not suddenly stop taking (or accidentally run out of) this medication. It can cause a hypertensive rebound, with potentially dangerous cardiovascular results.

Propranolol is a beta-blocker used for hypertension that can also treat the physical symptoms of anxiety, including the akathisia caused by other psychiatric medications. It is an excellent medication when your client has predominantly what is called psychomotor agitation: sweaty palms, racing heartbeat, hyperventilation, and a sense of impending doom. Taking propranolol can both treat and prevent this type of anxiety. However, it does not affect the cognitive symptoms of anxiety, so it will not decrease rumination or worry. Propranolol has also been shown to decrease the development of PTSD, as it can treat the arousal resulting from sudden exposure to trauma without interfering with the brain's ability to process the event (unlike benzodiazepines, which do interfere with this process). It is also not addicting. Adversely, propranolol can drop blood pressure, so be sure to ask your client if they are getting dizzy or experiencing falls. If so, contact their prescriber, who will need to either drop the dose or discontinue the medication.

Case Example

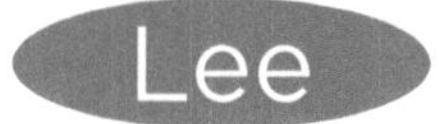

Lee was a 28-year-old man who was newly sober. He was taking 60 mg of Prozac (fluoxetine) for major depressive disorder, which was in remission, but he was now acutely anxious after having stopped drinking alcohol. He came into session wringing his hands, talking loudly, and insisting "something be done" about his anxiety. He wanted to continue taking Prozac but said, "I just need something *now* to help me."

Although he was committed to his sobriety, he was worried he might resume drinking because "these nerves are driving me nuts." He agreed on a trial of hydroxyzine (25 to 50 mg up to three times a day) for a short time to assist him with getting through these "rough days."

He found he did best with 25 mg in the morning and 50 mg at night, and after a few weeks, he no longer needed the medication and stopped it. He continued the Prozac throughout, and his depressive symptoms stayed in remission.

Case Example

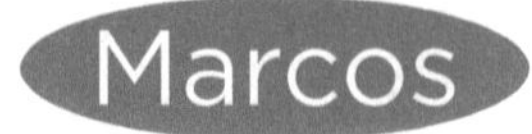

Marcos is a 50-year-old man with severe, debilitating social phobia. He was previously homeless for several years because he often did not come to appointments or even answer his phone, even when he knew it was critical to keeping his housing. He has a history of alcohol use disorder, which is currently in remission, but he continues to struggle with the urge to drink when his heightened anxiety becomes "intolerable."

Currently, he ventures out in public only to the grocery store (late at night) and, sometimes, to see me. He denies being suicidal but says he is "miserable." He has seen innumerable other counselors and has been tried on many SSRIs, SNRIs, and benzodiazepines—all with minimal effect.

He had recently hoped to start a specialty anxiety treatment program involving exposure therapy but became frustrated by the confusing intake process and gave up. I decided to start him on a trial of a tricyclic (nortriptyline), which he is slowly increasing, as well as Seroquel (quetiapine) at bedtime.

He reported that the Seroquel is helping and said, "At least I get relief when I sleep now." After the tricyclic is at a therapeutic dose, he may be able to taper off the Seroquel.

Antihistamines for Anxiety

Antihistamines can also play a role in treating immediate anxiety symptoms. The most commonly used agent is hydroxyzine, which requires a prescription. Unlike Benadryl (diphenhydramine), hydroxyzine is thought to interact with certain serotonin receptors to produce a mild anti-anxiety effect. Generally, clients either find it helpful or don't like it at all. Clients who have recently stopped using substances find that hydroxyzine is particularly helpful in providing immediate relief from anxiety symptoms while other portions of their recovery plan (e.g., antidepressant medication, psychotherapy) get underway. Again, the dose your client finds helpful is highly variable. Some clients may find that 25 mg at bedtime is effective, while others may require 50 mg to even 100 mg multiple times daily. Hydroxyzine is not habit-forming, but it can cause dry mouth and sedation.

Atypical Antipsychotics for Anxiety

Atypical antipsychotics can be useful when treating severe anxiety disorders, both in terms of their ability to augment other agents and to provide anti-anxiety relief on their own. These agents should not be the first choice of medication because of their potential for weight gain, metabolic adversities, akathisia, and dystonia. Therefore, they should be reserved for the management of life-impairing anxiety symptoms when other agents have failed.

BuSpar

Finally, a unique agent for treating anxiety is BuSpar, though it is only effective with generalized anxiety disorder. It does not work with social anxiety or panic disorder. It is typically prescribed with twice-daily dosing, as some clients have nausea on a once-a-day dose, which makes it more difficult for clients to take. It also tends to be under-dosed. Primary care providers tend to prescribe 10 mg twice a day, but very few clients get better at this dose and frequently need 30-45 mg daily. If your client is prescribed this agent, make sure they know it will take weeks to months to work—as opposed to anti-anxiety medication that works right away—so they shouldn't give up on it after a week or two.

Measuring Change in Anxiety

The Generalized Anxiety Disorder 7-Item Scale (GAD-7) is a valid self-report tool for measuring change in generalized anxiety disorder that can be completed quickly and is readily available online. The Panic Disorder Severity Scale is another valid self-report tool for measuring change, although it is cumbersome in that while there are only nine items, each has multiple choices with significant reading involved. Clients who cannot read or who read poorly might respond easier to a chart that allows them to check their levels of impairment across the questions, similar to the GAD-7 or PHQ-9. Finally, the PTSD Checklist for *DSM-5* (PCL-5) is easy to complete and valid for measuring severity and change in PTSD. These tools give you the data you need to determine if treatment is working and how much progress is being made, or if you need to modify your treatment plan. This, in turn, increases the effectiveness of care and improves outcomes.

Vulnerable Populations

Pregnant Women

Like mood disorders, anxiety can worsen during pregnancy and the postpartum period. The postpartum period in particular can be a time of increased vulnerability to develop anxiety given the major life changes that having a newborn brings. So assess for anxiety regularly, and communicate those findings with your client's psychiatric prescriber, as well as the health care provider managing the pregnancy. Anxiety, like depression, is not good for the developing fetus. If medication is warranted, the SSRIs and tricyclics are considered reasonable, relatively safe options for treatment of anxiety during pregnancy.

However, caution should be taken regarding the use of benzodiazepines during pregnancy. If you have a client who becomes pregnant while taking benzodiazepines, she needs to talk with her women's health care provider. Caution your client against suddenly stopping the benzodiazepine, as doing so is harmful and can cause a resurgence in anxiety symptoms. In addition, your client's provider may prefer that she stay on medication. If not, they will tell your client how to taper off. Never suddenly discontinue benzodiazepines.

Youth

SSRIs are the medication of choice when it comes to treating anxiety in youth, as these medications are even more effective for adolescents than they are for adults. However, the dose must be extremely small with younger clients (ten percent of the adult starting dose) to prevent akathisia and corresponding suicidality.

When left untreated, anxiety in children and adolescents can contribute to conflicts at home, school failure, and the development of a sense of being unable to manage the challenges of life. These clients may "give up" when activities and school and relationships get hard. These difficulties all contribute to suicidality. If your client is struggling in this manner, do a deep dive and assess for an anxiety disorder.

Older Adults

Anxiety disorders tend to attenuate in older adults, although anxiety and agitation are often seen in episodes of depression and dementia syndromes. If you have an older client struggling with anxiety, take time to problem solve the sources of this anxiety. Is it a fear resulting from a change in their environment? Does your client feel they are in danger? Or do they feel safe? What about recent losses? Identifying and addressing psychosocial losses and changes is highly effective for decreasing anxiety (and treating depression as well).

If your client needs medication, SSRIs are the treatment of choice for older adults, with the exception of Paxil, which is highly anticholinergic and increases the risk of memory impairment and falls (and resulting fractures). SSRIs are the preferred medication option because it is the only class of antidepressants that does not affect norepinephrine. Norepinephrine can impact cardiac rhythm, which is a frequent medical concern for older adults. This is why tricyclic antidepressants are contraindicated in older adults, with the exception of an ultra-low dose of doxepin (< 6 mg) for treating insomnia (Markota et al., 2016). And remember: Benzodiazepines carry risk of memory impairment, cognitive dysfunction, and increased falls, so these medications should be avoided when treating anxiety in older adults (American Geriatrics Society Beers Criteria Update Expert Panel, 2019).

Co-occurring Substance Use Disorders

Accumulating evidence has changed the expectation that clients must be clean and sober before receiving treatment for anxiety. Previously, clients were expected to be in recovery for three, and sometimes even six, months prior to evaluation and treatment. However, this perspective has shifted to one in which it is preferable to concurrently treat both conditions.

The SSRIs are the safest medications for clients with a co-occurring substance use disorder, though clients will need to be started at an ultra-low dose (ten percent of the usual starting dose) to prevent akathisia, which clients with a substance use history are exquisitely sensitive to. If clients have significant liver damage secondary to substance use, they may be limited to an even lower dose. In this situation, the medication impacts the brain the same way that it would in a client without liver damage, so that a low dose can be effective. Be sure to help your client understand even though the dose is lower, it may be the right dose—and the effective dose—for them. BuSpar (buspirone) and gabapentin can also be effective medications, though gabapentin should not be prescribed to clients with opiate use disorder, as it increases sedation and the feeling of being "high."

Of the other antidepressants, Cymbalta (duloxetine) increases the risk of liver failure in clients with a current or past alcohol use disorder, so it should be avoided. Tricyclic antidepressants should also be avoided due to their potential for overdose, which is a particular concern among clients who have a history of impulsive substance use behavior. Additionally, tricyclics can cause heart rhythm abnormalities among clients with stimulant use disorder. They also increase the risk of having a seizure if your client stops drinking, as does Wellbutrin (bupropion), so both of these medications should be avoided for clients with an alcohol use disorder.

Finally, benzodiazepines are contraindicated for clients with a current substance use disorder and must be used with extreme caution with clients who are sober but have a history of substance use. If you recall, benzodiazepines combined with alcohol or opiates can cause respiratory depression and death. Therefore, these agents may be reasonable only when your client **(1)** has been clean and sober for over a year, **(2)** has tried other agents and psychotherapies, **(3)** has a life-impairing anxiety disorder, and **(4)** is willing to work closely with you and their prescriber, including monitoring for substance use via urine drug screens (Posternak & Mueller, 2001).

Conclusion

Like many other mood disorders, anxiety is a very common, disabling, and treatable condition. Although evidence-based psychotherapy is the treatment of choice, there are a variety of medication options that can augment psychotherapy—and medication may indeed be critical to facilitate recovery from life-impairing anxiety. With the possible exception of benzodiazepines, medications work well in conjunction with therapy, particularly with CBT, which doubles or triples the positive outcomes of treatment, even in older adults, compared to medication alone (Marra et al., 2015).

It is also important to recognize and treat anxiety when it is comorbid with other mood or psychotic disorders, as doing so improves client outcomes. At times, anxiety is so intertwined with depression that when one condition worsens, so does the other. The good news is that treating one disorder often treats the other as well. Therefore, even if anxiety is not your client's top worry, don't overlook it. It may be key to treating many concerns.

Chapter 6

Complementary and Alternative Medication

Although prescription medication is often the first type of medication that comes to mind when people think of standard medical care, it is not the only treatment option. Complementary and alternative medication (CAM) is another option that can be used instead of, or in conjunction with, more mainstream approaches to medication. As a whole, CAM refers to any type of product or practice that is not considered under the umbrella of conventional medical care.

There are many situations when the use of CAMs is an excellent resource, such as when a client is reluctant to see a prescriber or is fearful of taking prescribed medications. Or, it can be helpful when a client is frustrated with side effects, as CAMs have fewer side effects and very few drug interactions. For example, if a client is taking Zoloft (sertraline) for mild to moderate depression but is unable to tolerate the jitteriness, switching over to a CAM may be a great choice. One caveat: Don't trade a decrease in side effects for a loss of effectiveness. Think effectiveness first, and the minimization of adverse effects second.

Different types of CAMs can also be particularly helpful for clients who have mild to moderate depression (e.g., a PHQ-9 score at or below 19). Many of these agents work equally as well as prescription antidepressants, though they do not work for severe depression. When a client with depression has improved on prescription medication but is still exhibiting residual symptoms, CAMs can also augment the effects of the antidepressant and allow them to achieve full remission. With a few exceptions, which are noted in this chapter, CAMs can be taken at the same time as prescription medication. Finally, CAMs offer treatment for some conditions, notably trichotillomania, for which there is no effective prescription option.

CAMs fall into several categories, which include antioxidants, herbal agents, hormones, amino acids and their precursors, and vitamins. This chapter does not provide an exhaustive list regarding each of these different categories, but it does discuss specific agents that have undergone rigorous testing and proven effective for the conditions discussed in this book. Some of these agents are listed in the next table. For readers interested in additional information regarding CAMs, the book *Complementary and Integrative Treatments in Psychiatric Practice* (Gerbarg, 2019) is an excellent reference.

Effective Complementary and Alternative Medications

Name	Uses	Dose
Rhodiola rosea	Mild to moderate depression; Anxiety; Akathisia; Dystonia	300-800 mg daily; Use formulations with 3% rosavins
Valerian	Anxiety; Insomnia	200-300 mg in the morning; 450 mg at bedtime
St. John's wort	Mild to moderate depression	300-800 mg daily; Cannot be taken with prescription antidepressants
SAM-e	Mild to moderate depression	800-2400 mg daily
N-acetylcysteine (NAC)	Bipolar depression; OCD; Akathisia; Trichotillomania	1200-2400 mg daily
L-tryptophan	Premenstrual dysphoric disorder (PMDD); Augmentation of antidepressants	300 mg for the treatment of PMDD; Up to 6,000 mg daily for the treatment of depression
Omega-3 fatty acids	Augmentation of antidepressants	1,000 to 2,000 mg daily with > 60% EPA
Melatonin	Insomnia	0.5 mg to 15 mg two hours before bedtime; Extended-release formulation promotes staying asleep

In the sections that follow, you'll find more specific information regarding these different types of CAMs, including which clients are likely good candidates, what conditions they can treat, and how they work well with prescription medications. CAM is not regulated by the FDA, nor is it held to the same standards for purity and manufacturing as prescribed medications, so—with a few exceptions—I do not recommend suggesting these agents to vulnerable clients. If they are used at all with vulnerable populations, be sure to recommend high-quality manufacturers.

Herbal Agents

Rhodiola rosea is an herb found at high altitudes in Europe and Asia with proven effectiveness for mild to moderate depression and generalized anxiety disorder in randomized controlled trials (Bystritsky et al., 2008; Darbinyan et al., 2007). Its efficacy is equivalent to that of an SSRI for clients with mild to moderate depression but not those with moderate to severe depression, so make sure to help clients with more significant depression connect to a prescriber. Additionally, there are reports of rhodiola rosea effectively treating anxiety, cognitive slowing, and depression in postmenopausal women (Gerbarg, 2019). It also prevents altitude sickness and treats impotence.

Rhodiola rosea is considered an "adaptogen" in that it promotes resilience to chemical, biological, and physical stress. It is possible this adaptogen is also neuroprotective (Muskin, Gerbarg, & Brown, 2013) and may decrease the akathisia and dystonia side effects from psychiatric medications. It has both anti-inflammatory and antioxidant properties. Side effects are rare, and it's relatively inexpensive. Your client can use it alone, or in combination with prescription antidepressants or other prescription psychiatric medication, as there are no drug interactions of concern. When a client responds well to an antidepressant but exhibits only a partial treatment response, adding rhodiola rosea can augment the medication and help them achieve full remission.

It is recommended that clients take rhodiola rosea on an empty stomach. It is generally well-tolerated, and the most common complaint is a mild feeling of stimulation or being energized. Because it is slightly stimulating, clients may prefer taking it in the morning instead of at bedtime. When combined with large amounts of caffeine, it can also cause rapid heart rate. It has some potential for triggering a hypomanic episode in clients with bipolar disorders. The effective dose is 300 mg daily to twice daily, with a maximum dose of 800 mg. The brand chosen should have three percent rosavins.

Valerian is another type of herb that has been used since ancient Greece and Roman times for insomnia and anxiety. It promotes GABA, which is the calming neurotransmitter. It does not cause a daytime "hangover," so it may be appealing for some clients. It is proven safe with youth, older adults, and pregnant women. For insomnia, the dose is 450-600 mg taken two hours before bed. Alert your client that they need to take it every night for at least two weeks for full effectiveness. Adding a morning dose of 250-300 mg also makes it effective for generalized anxiety disorder.

St. John's wort is another herbal medication that is equally as effective as prescription antidepressants in the treatment of mild to moderate major depression. It may also reduce cytokines, which are implicated in the inflammatory process connected to bipolar disorders. As discussed in Chapter 2, St. John's wort is a mild SSRI, so it should not be taken with prescription antidepressants to avoid serious serotonin syndrome. In addition, alert your client that St. John's wort decreases the effectiveness of oral contraceptives. The effective dose is 300-1800 mg daily, usually split across two doses. Make sure that clients do not use a very low-cost version, as its poor potency will make it ineffective.

Finally, ***kava***, which functions as a plant-based muscle relaxant, is effective for anxiety, but there are several concerns regarding its safety—which is why it is not included in the table. It can cause liver impairment and failure at any dose, even after taking it for one month. As a result, many countries have limited or discontinued its availability. It can also be addictive for some clients.

Amino Acids

SAM-e (or S-adenosylmethionine) is an amino acid precursor that has demonstrated its effectiveness in treating mild to moderate depression across several double-blind randomized controlled studies (Muskin et al., 2013; Sharma et al., 2017). Its efficacy is similar to that of the SSRIs and tricyclics—and is associated with fewer adverse effects. It may also help with cognitive function after brain injury. In addition to its independent treatment effect, SAM-e can be used to augment prescription antidepressants when they are not working or have only resulted in a partial treatment response. It also helps restore antidepressant benefit when these medications have quit working (the so-called "Prozac poop-out"). Not commonly, but at times, the combination of an SSRI and SAM-e can trigger anxiety. It is contraindicated for clients with bipolar disorders for its potential to induce hypomania, though this risk is less than with antidepressants.

The usual starting dose is 200-400 mg, with clients gradually increasing the dose every few days until they achieve 800-1600 mg daily. If that is not effective, it can be titrated to a maximum dose of 2400 mg daily. It should be taken on an empty stomach first thing in the morning, with a second dose taken before lunch, at least a half an hour before eating. It is not recommended to take SAM-e after mid-day given its stimulating effect, which can interfere with sleep. Although there are no controlled studies with children or adolescents, there are some case reports that SAM-e is effective in youth with a dose of 200-600 mg daily. SAM-e is also safe to use with liver disease and may support liver function. The maximum dose with liver disease is 1200 mg daily.

SAM-e tends to be more expensive, but low-quality SAM-e loses its potency. Because SAM-e works in conjunction with B12 and folate, clients can obtain a similar benefit with a lower dose by combining it with these supplements, which are inexpensive. SAM-e tablets should also be individually packaged to prevent oxidation.

For many clients, SAM-e is initially challenging to take due to nausea and vomiting. The use of enteric-coated tables can help decrease nausea, as can slowly increasing the dose instead of starting at the full therapeutic dose. SAM-e can cause anxiety during the titration process until clients acclimate to the medication, so it is important to slow down the increases in dose if this occurs. It does not cause weight gain.

NAC (n-acetylcysteine) is an antioxidant that has long been used in emergency settings for the treatment of Tylenol (acetaminophen) overdoses. However, studies have tested its effectiveness in treating many other medical issues (such as chronic obstructive pulmonary disease, kidney disease, and HIV), as well as many psychiatric disorders, including autism spectrum disorders and neurocognitive disorders (Gerbarg, 2019). It is particularly effective in treating trichotillomania and skin picking disorder, for which there are no effective prescription medications. There are also multiple randomized controlled trials demonstrating that it can be used as an augment to Risperdal to reduce irritability in autism spectrum disorders (Nikoo et al., 2015). In addition, it reduces akathisia and improves overall global functioning in clients with schizophrenia. Multiple studies show its efficacy in treating depressive episodes in bipolar disorders (Berk et al., 2008), with less data supporting its use in treating major depressive disorder. It is also effective for treatment-resistant OCD (Gerbarg, 2019).

Dosing for these mental health indications is 1200 mg once to twice daily. It takes up to three months for clients to see its full effect. NAC is well tolerated, does not cause weight gain, has no drug interactions, and is relatively inexpensive. However, it can cause agitation or (hypo)mania in clients with bipolar disorders, similar to antidepressants but at a much less frequent rate. Monitor clients regularly and encourage them to talk over any symptoms they are having with their prescriber.

Case Example

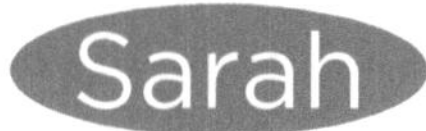

Sarah, who was 33 years old, was in a depressive episode of her bipolar I disorder—again. Years ago, she had become manic on Zoloft (sertraline) and knew never to take it again. She had also been on Lamictal (lamotrigine) without benefit.

Currently, she was on lithium, and her dose was solidly therapeutic at 0.8 mEq/L. However, she was spending an increasing amount of days in bed and requested help.

We discussed options and decided on a trial of N-acetylcysteine (NAC). She continued her lithium as well. Two weeks later, she reported having had to stop the NAC because she felt "exactly like I did when I took Zoloft. It scared me!"

L-tryptophan is an amino acid that is a precursor to tryptophan and serotonin. It works for the treatment of premenstrual dysphoric disorder (PMDD) at 300 mg per day and mild to moderate depression at 6,000 mg or 6 grams daily. It also has some (less robust) evidence regarding its ability to augment the effect of antidepressants at doses of 300 mg a day. The most common adverse effects with L-tryptophan include gastrointestinal distress, such as nausea, vomiting, cramping, and diarrhea.

Omega-3 fatty acids (fish oil) are another type of CAM that can be helpful with depression. The best evidence for omega-3 fatty acids is for augmenting the effect of antidepressants in major depression and stabilizing mood in bipolar disorders. There is also evidence they can decrease the risk of developing schizophrenia following first-episode psychosis among individuals at extremely high risk for the disorder (Amminger et al., 2010; Pawelczyk, 2016). The suggested dose is 1,000 to 2,000mg of omega-3 fatty acids daily, with a supplement that contains at least 60 percent eicosapentaenoic acid (EPA) (Gerbarg, 2019). The fish oil milligram is not the same as the omega-3 fatty acid milligram. The risks of use are very low, so it is often recommended in spite of mixed evidence, and it also conveys a heart health benefit.

Finally, ***melatonin*** can be helpful with insomnia, which is a common symptom of many psychiatric disorders and is a side effect of many prescription medications as well. Melatonin is a natural hormone produced by the pineal gland in the brain that is exclusively released in complete darkness. Melatonin supplements are effective for improving the onset and duration of sleep and have no short- or long-term adverse effects (Xie et al., 2017). The dosage can range from 0.5 mg to even 15 mg nightly. It is best taken a few hours prior to bedtime to allow the natural hormone to create sleepiness. For clients who have trouble staying asleep, the use of an extended-release formulation has also proven effective. Be sure to alert your client to take the medication several hours before bed, not at bedtime.

Conclusion

The use of CAMs is a welcome addition to the "regular" prescribed medication approach. I first consider these agents when I know there are effective over-the-counter options for what my client is experiencing. Effectiveness is always the first consideration. In addition, CAMs can be an excellent option for clients who do not want prescription medication, who do not want to see a prescriber, or who have no access to a prescriber. They also work well for clients struggling with adverse effects from prescription medication since they tend to have less side effects. Finally, these are a good option for clients who have gotten somewhat better on prescription medication but have not achieved full remission, as CAMs can safely serve as an augmenting agent.

Communicate with your client's prescriber if they are already on psychiatric medication and are thinking about CAMs. Although these are over-the-counter medications, you should never tell your client to simply start taking one of these agents. Rather, your role is to provide information about these agents as options for treatment and to encourage your client to discuss any questions with their psychiatric or other health care provider.

Chapter 7

———

Going Forward

It is an exciting time to be working in this field. We are on the cusp of new medication approaches, such as ketamine for depression, and new understandings, such as the contributions of inflammation and other medical conditions to the brain and mental illnesses. Indeed, we are beginning to see these conditions not just as "mental" illnesses but as multi-systemic conditions. We are growing our understanding of how to best treat depression, bipolar disorders, psychotic disorders, and anxiety—and you are part of it.

Therefore, this book has laid out a practical and adaptable framework, including specific strategies and tools, that enable you to become a full, active participant in helping your clients benefit from medications. But this is not the end. These ideas and strategies are meant to be a catalyst, an invitation if you will, to explore how you can build on this framework in a way that reflects your creativity and personal therapy style. I invite you to be curious about how the philosophical approach and practical strategies included here can work for different clients in your practice. How might you adapt these ideas in different ways to make your practice even more effective?

Clients benefit the most from treatment when we ground our work from a place of deep respect. Do not underestimate the power of working *with* them. When you understand their experiences, respect their concerns, communicate openly, and provide them with understandable information and real choices regarding psychiatric medication, good things happen. They become engaged and motivated to participate in the process. They become more likely to pursue medication when they need it. And they will be safer doing so, knowing they can talk with you about any problems that arise. They will be better equipped to make decisions about medications and understand what the specific agents are, how they work, and what to expect. By measuring change and communicating with their prescriber, you also create a pathway toward more seamless, effective care that ultimately improves treatment outcomes.

You are a vital, powerful resource in helping your clients reap the benefits and minimize the harm from psychiatric medication. Thank you for venturing forward on this journey. I hope you find this compendium of information and framework of strategies a useful toolbox, one you will return to over and over again.

Tools for Measuring Change

Tools for Depression

1. Patient Health Questionnaire (PHQ-9; Kroenke, Spitzer, & Williams, 2001): https://www.phqscreeners.com/

2. PHQ-9 for Adolescents (PHQ-9 A; Johnson, Harris, Spitzer, & Williams, 2002): https://www.uacap.org/uploads/3/2/5/0/3250432/phq-a.pdf

3. Center for Epidemiological Studies Depression Scale for Children (CES-DC; Fendrich, Weissman, & Warner, 1990): https://www.brightfutures.org/mentalhealth/pdf/professionals/bridges/ces_dc.pdf

4. Quick Inventory of Depressive Symptomatology (QIDS; Rush et al., 2003): https://eprovide.mapi-trust.org/instruments/quick-inventory-of-depressive-symptomatology

5. Geriatric Depression Scale (GDS; Yesavage et al., 1986): https://consultgeri.org/try-this/general-assessment/issue-4.pdf

6. Edinburgh Postnatal Depression Scale (Cox et al., 1987): https://www.fresno.ucsf.edu/pediatrics/downloads/edinburghscale.pdf

Tools for Bipolar Disorders

1. Altman Self-Rating Mania Scale (Altman, Hedeker, Peterson, & Davis, 1997) for detecting (hypo)mania: http://www.cqaimh.org/pdf/tool_asrm.pdf

2. PHQ-9 or QIDS (see above) for measuring depressive episodes.

3. Internal State Scale (Bauer et al., 1991) for measuring both (hypo)manic and depressive episodes: https://psychres.washington.edu/clinicaltools/internalstates_scale.pdf

4. Mood Disorder Questionnaire (MDQ; Hirschfield et al., 2000) for ruling out bipolar disorders: https://www.integration.samhsa.gov/images/res/MDQ.pdf

5. Mood Chart for measuring stability (See Appendix B: Resources for Clients)

Tools for Psychosis

1. Barnes Akathisia Rating Scale (BARS; Barnes, 1989): https://simpleandpractical. com/wp-content/uploads/2014/09/Barnes-Akathisia-Rating-Scale-BARS.pdf

2. Abnormal Involuntary Movement Scale (AIMS; Guy, 1976): https://www. aacap.org/App_Themes/AACAP/docs/member_resources/toolbox_for_ clinical_practice_and_outcomes/monitoring/AIMS.pdf

3. Use a 5-point Likert scale to measure the intensity of psychotic symptoms (0 = no symptoms; 5 = the worst the symptoms have ever been)

Tools for Anxiety

1. Generalized Anxiety Disorder 7-item Scale (GAD-7; Spitzer, Kroenke, Williams, & Löwe, 2006): http://www.phqscreeners.com/sites/g/files/ g10016261/f/201412/GAD-7_English.pdf

2. Panic Disorder Severity Rating Scale (Shear et al., 1997): http://www. goodmedicine.org.uk/files/panic,%20assessment%20pdss.pdf

3. PTSD Checklist for DSM-5 (PCL-5; Weathers et al., 2013): https://www.ptsd. va.gov/professional/assessment/documents/PCL5_Standard_form.PDF

Resources for Clients

General Resources

1. Medisafe® App (free): Provides reminders to take medication, displays pictures of pills to take, and alerts clients when they need a refill.

2. WILD 5 (Wellness Interventions for Life Demands): Provides low-cost, evidence-based manuals that break down wellness behaviors into manageable "chunks." These programs focus on nutrition, mindfulness, social connection, sleep, and exercise.

Depression Resources

Online Resources

1. Depression Bipolar Support Alliance (www.dbsalliance.org): Provides a wealth of information about mood disorders and medication. Clients can register to participate in the Wellness Tracker or the Wellness House, which includes "rooms" full of recovery and self-care ideas.

2. National Alliance on Mental Illness (www.nami.org): Provides the latest facts, statistics, and research advances on different types of mental health conditions.

3. National Council of Behavioral Health (www.thenationalcouncil.org): Provides inspiring stories of treatment success.

4. Recovery International (recoveryinternational.org): Using cognitive-behavioral methods, this organization seeks to augment psychotherapy by helping people with depression identify triggers and cognitive errors, focusing primarily on anger/blame and worthlessness/self-blame. Provides online, phone, chat, in-person, and Facebook meetings worldwide.

App Resources

1. Daylio (free): Helps client rate their mood with smiling to frowning faces and allows them to connect their mood with their activity level. Data is displayed

graphically so clients can see the relationship between their mood and activity across time. It can also give them reminders to journal or engage in self-care. The app's one-tap journaling function allows clients to record their experiences—with no writing required.

2. Youper® AI (free): Provides an "emotional health assistant" with whom clients can talk back and forth, with a focus on gaining perspective on troubling events.

3. What's Up?® (free): By combining the concepts of both CBT and acceptance and commitment therapy, this app provides mood charting, a diary function, grounding exercises, and breathing techniques.

4. Depression CBT Self-Help (free): This audio mood management app can help clients manage stressful daily situations (e.g., commuting). It also helps evaluate their mood and enhance their motivation through a point system.

5. My3 (free): This teen app for suicide prevention incorporates the principles of evidence-based safety planning. Using just one tap, clients can easily contact their three identified supports when they need help. It also has a one-tap function for professional suicide prevention and another tap for 911.

6. Code Blue (free): Similar to My3, this app is designed for teens dealing with depression, suicidality, or bullying. Clients input their supports, and with one tap they are able to alert their support group. The app's functionality also provides the client's location, so supports can know where to find the client and let the client know they're coming.

7. notOK® (free): Similar to My3 and Code Blue, this app allows clients to identify who their support group is (the "crew"), and then one tap alerts the crew that the client needs support.

Bipolar Resources

Online Resources

1. bp Magazine and bpHope.com: bp Magazine is a quarterly magazine with many in-depth articles about living life with bipolar disorders (print $19.95; digital $9.95). The online version (www.bphope.com) provides a free weekly email that is written by people living life with bipolar disorders. Highly recommended.

2. Depression Bipolar Support Alliance (www.dbsalliance.org): This is an excellent resource for clients to learn more about bipolar disorders, connect with others living with bipolar disorders, and learn self-care strategies. The "Facing Us Clubhouse" has a wellness tracker, resources, and strategies for managing life with bipolar disorders.

3. PsychEducation (psychEducation.org): This non-profit website provides extensive information about bipolar disorders.

4. MoodNetwork (www.moodnetwork.org): Developed by Massachusetts General Hospital, this website provides information on bipolar disorders, resources, and crisis contacts.

App Resources

1. eMoods Bipolar Mood Tracker (free): This mood charting app is one of the few apps that includes irritable mood, elevated mood, and depression on the continuum. Many apps for depression only have "feeling good" or "feeling great" as the highest descriptor, which is not useful for clients with bipolar disorders. The app has the capacity to graph results and track other behaviors in addition to mood.

2. My3 (free)

3. Code Blue (free)

4. notOK (free)

Additional Resources

1. Monthly Mood Chart: A simplified monthly mood chart is provided on the next page, but there are also many complex versions online. Be careful not to use charts that list feeling "fine" at the top of the scale.

Monthly Mood Chart

	1	2	3	4	5	6	7	8	9	10	11	12	13	14	15	16	17	18	19	20	21	22	23	24	25	26	27	28	29	30	31
(Hypo)mania: Increased energy, Racing thoughts																															
Euthymic: Enjoying life, Feeling good																															
Depressed: Low energy, Feeling sluggish																															

Psychosis

Online Resources

1. National Alliance on Mental Illness (www.nami.org): Provides support groups and advocacy efforts for people with serious mental illnesses.

2. Schizophrenia and Related Disorders Alliance of America (www.sardaa.org): SARDAA provides peer support groups and weekly conference calls to help improve the lives of individuals with psychotic disorders. It promotes hope with stories of recovery and also provides information and resources regarding psychotic disorders.

App Resources

1. SARDAA Health Storylines (free): This app was created by SARDAA for individuals with schizophrenia and related disorders. It is a tool that allows clients to track their symptoms, set medication reminders, keep track of appointments, journal about their experiences, and connect with others experiencing psychotic disorders.

Additional Resources

1. Small meals and snack ideas (about 350 kcal) for use with Latuda:

Open-faced Peanut Butter Banana Sandwich		Chips and Dip	
	Calories		Calories
1 slice of whole wheat bread	70	¼ cup of salsa	30
2 tbsp of peanut butter	190	¼ medium avocado	70
1 banana	105	2 oz (about 20) tortilla chips	275
Total	365	Total	375
Apple, Cheese, Crackers, and Milk or Juice		**Avocado Toast with Cheese**	
	Calories		Calories
1 medium apple	95	1 slice of whole wheat bread	70
1 oz cheese	100	½ medium avocado	140
6 whole wheat crackers	120	1 oz cheese	100
½ cup of skim milk or juice	45-60	½ cup of juice	45
Total	350-375	Total	355

Rice and Beans	Calories	Yogurt, Granola, and Fruit	Calories
½ cup of cooked brown rice	100	6 oz container of nonfat yogurt	80
½ can of black beans	171	½ cup of low-fat granola	210
1 oz shredded cheese	100	1 cup of blueberries	80
Total	371	Total	360
Chips and Juice	Calories	**Oreos and Milk**	Calories
1 snack bag of potato chips	160	5 Oreos	268
1 bottle of orange juice	220	1 cup of low-fat or skim milk	90-120
Total	380	Total	358-388
Turkey Sandwich	Calories	**Cup of Noodles and Egg**	Calories
2 slices of whole wheat bread	140	1 vegetable Cup Noodles®	290
2 tbsp of mustard	20	1 hardboiled egg	80
1 thin slice of cheese	100		
3 slices of turkey	90		
Total	350	Total	370

Anxiety Disorders

Online Resources

1. Recovery International (recoveryinternational.org)

App Resources

1. CALM® (free): This awarding-winning app provides adult "sleep stories," mindfulness meditations, and strategies to manage anxiety and stress. The premium version ($59) opens up more sleep stories and more in-depth "masterclass" material.

2. Headspace® (free): This app provides guided meditations led by a former monk on issues related to sleep, happiness, productivity, mindful use of technology, and other topics. Clients can use the app to track their time in mindfulness training and invite friends to join in with them.

3. Rootd (free): This female-led app focuses on decreasing panic attacks. It provides mindfulness exercises and step-by-step guides on strategies to reduce panic, such as deep breathing. It also has an emergency contact button that

allows clients to contact a support person in the event of a panic attack. It tracks the number of panic attacks clients have overcome, as well as the number of completed lessons.

4. Stop, Breathe & Think® (free): This app provides short, guided meditations determined by the mood selected. It also provides ideas for acupressure and yoga, as well as deep breathing exercises and visualizations to "tame" anxiety. The app also allows clients to track their progress.

5. Colorfy® (free): This digital, adult coloring book app uses distraction to decrease anxiety. Clients can choose from a selection of images and mandalas, or they can upload their own sketches to color.

6. DARE—Break Free from Anxiety (free): This app focuses on helping clients overcome their fears, anxiety, panic, worry, or insomnia. It contains audio recordings to help clients increase distress tolerance rather than avoiding anxiety.

Appendix C

Additional Resources for You

Carlat, D. (Ed.). *The Carlat psychiatry report*. Monthly publication. Newburyport, MA: Carlat Publishing. (Available at www.thecarlatreport.com)

Goldberg, J., & Ernst, C. (2019). *Managing the side effects of psychotropic medications* (Rev. ed.). Washington, DC: American Psychiatric Press.

Jordan, T. (Ed.). (2019). *Psychiatry practice boosters* (2nd ed.). Newburyport, MA: Carlat Publishing.

Meyer, J. S., & Quenzer, L.F. (2018). *Psychopharmacology: Drugs, the brain and behavior* (3rd ed.). Sunderland, MA: Sinauer Associates.

Schmacher, J., & Madson, M. B. (2015). *Fundamentals of motivational interviewing: Tips and strategies for addressing common clinical challenges*. New York: Oxford University Press.

Shea, S. C. (2018). *The medication interest model: How to talk with patients about their medications* (2nd ed). Philadelphia: Wolters Kluwer.

Stahl, S. (2013). *Stahl's essentials of psychopharmacology: Neuroscientific basis and practical applications* (4th ed.). New York: Cambridge University Press.

Stahl, S. (2017). *The prescriber's guide: Stahl's essential psychopharmacology* (6th ed.). New York: Cambridge University Press.

References

Abé, C., Ekman, C. J., Sellgren, C., Petrovic, P., Ingvar, M., & Landén, M. (2015). Manic episodes are related to changes in frontal cortex: A longitudinal neuroimaging study of bipolar disorder 1. *Brain, 138*(11), 3440–3448.

Ahmed, S., Bachu, R., Kotapati, P., Adnan, M., Ahmed, R., Farooq, U., … Begum, G. (2019). Use of gabapentin in the treatment of substance use and psychiatric disorders: A systematic review. *Frontiers in Psychiatry, 10,* 228.

Altman, E. G., Hedeker, D., Peterson, J. L., & Davis, J. M. (1997). The Altman Self-Rating Mania Scale. *Biological Psychiatry, 42*(10), 948–955.

American Geriatrics Society Beers Criteria® Update Expert Panel. (2019). American Geriatrics Society 2019 updated AGS Beers Criteria® for potentially inappropriate medication use in older adults. *Journal of the American Geriatrics Society, 67*(4), 674–694.

American Psychiatric Association. (2013). *Diagnostic and statistical manual of mental disorders* (5th ed.). Arlington, VA: Author.

Amminger, G. P., Schäfer, M. R., Papageorgiou, K., Klier, C. M., Cotton, S. M., Harrigan, S. M., … Berger, G. E. (2010). Long-chain omega-3 fatty acids for indicated prevention of psychotic disorders: A randomized, placebo-controlled trial. *Archives of General Psychiatry, 67*(2), 146–154.

Antosik-Wójcińska, A., Stefanowski, B., & Święcicki, Ł. (2015). Efficacy and safety of antidepressants' use in the treatment of depressive episodes in bipolar disorder—review of research. *Psychiatra Polska, 49*(6), 1223–1239.

Bandelow, B., & Michaelis, S. (2015). Epidemiology of anxiety disorders in the 21st century. *Dialogues in Clinical Neuroscience, 17*(3), 327–335.

Barnes, T. R. (1989). A rating scale for drug-induced akathisia. *The British Journal of Psychiatry, 154*(5), 672–676.

Bauer, M. S., Crits-Christoph, P., Ball, W. A., Dewees, E., McAllister, T., Alahi, P., … Whybrow, P. C. (1991). Independent assessment of manic and depressive symptoms by self-rating: Scale characteristics and implications for the study of mania. *Archives of General Psychiatry, 48*(9), 807–812.

Bauer, M. S., Miller, C. J., Li, M., Bajor, L. A., & Lee, A. (2016). A population-based study of the comparative effectiveness of second-generation antipsychotics vs. older antimanic agents in bipolar disorder. *Bipolar Disorders, 18*(6), 481–489.

Berk, M., Copolov, D. L., Dean, O., Lu, K., Jeavons, S., Schapkaitz, I., … Bush, A. I. (2008). N-acetylcysteine for depressive symptoms in bipolar disorder—a double-blind randomized placebo-controlled trial. *Biological Psychiatry, 64*(6), 468–475.

Bighelli, I., Trespidi, C., Castellazzi, M., Cipriani, A., Furukawa, T. A., Girlanda, F., … Barbui, C. (2016). Antidepressants and benzodiazepines for panic disorder in adults. *Cochrane Database of Systematic Reviews, 9,* No. CD011567.

Bjerre, L. M., Farrell, B., Hogel, M., Graham, L., Lemay, G., McCarthy, L., … Welch, V. (2018). Deprescribing antipsychotics for behavioural and psychological symptoms of dementia and insomnia: Evidence-based clinical practice guideline. *Canadian Family Physician, 64*(1), 17–27.

Brown, M. T., & Bussell, J. K. (2011). Medication adherence: WHO cares? *Mayo Clinic Proceedings, 86*(4), 304–314.

Bystritsky, A., Kerwin, L., & Feusner, J. D. (2008). A pilot study of Rhodiola rosea (Rhodax®) for generalized anxiety disorder (GAD). *The Journal of Alternative and Complementary Medicine, 14*(2), 175–180.

Calabrese, J. R., Shelton, M. D., Rapport, D. J., Kujawa, M., Kimmel, S. E., & Caban, S. (2001). Current research on rapid cycling bipolar disorder and its treatment. *Journal of Affective Disorders, 67*(1-3), 241–255.

Cipriani, A., Reid, K., Young, A. H., Macritchie, K., & Geddes, J. (2013). Valproic acid, valproate and divalproex in the maintenance treatment of bipolar disorder. *Cochrane Database of Systematic Reviews,* (10), CD003196.

Cohen, L. S., Altshuler, L. L., Harlow, B. L., Nonacs, R., Newport, D. J., Viguera, A. C., … Loughead, A. (2006). Relapse of major depression during pregnancy in women who maintain or discontinue antidepressant treatment. *JAMA, 295*(5), 499–507.

Cohen, M. J., Meador, K. J., May, R., Loblein, H., Conrad, T., Baker, G. A., … Liporace, J. D. (2019). Fetal antiepileptic drug exposure and learning and memory functioning at 6 years of age: The NEAD prospective observational study. *Epilepsy & Behavior, 92*, 154–164.

Cook, J. A., Copeland, M. E., Jonikas, J. A., Hamilton, M. M., Razzano, L. A., Grey, D. D., … Boyd, S. (2012). Results of a randomized controlled trial of mental illness self-management using Wellness Recovery Action Planning. *Schizophrenia Bulletin, 38*(4), 881–891.

Cox, J. L., Holden, J. M., & Sagovsky, R. (1987). Detection of postnatal depression: Development of the 10-item Edinburgh Postnatal Depression Scale. *British Journal of Psychiatry, 150*, 782–786.

Darbinyan, V., Aslanyan, G., Amroyan, E., Gabrielyan, E., Malmström, C., & Panossian, A. (2007). Clinical trial of Rhodiola rosea L. extract SHR-5 in the treatment of mild to moderate depression. *Nordic Journal of Psychiatry, 61*(5), 343–348.

Felitti, V. J., Anda, R. F., Nordenberg, D., Williamson, D. F., Spitz, A. M., Edwards, V., & Marks, J. S. (1998). Relationship of childhood abuse and household dysfunction to many of the leading causes of death in adults: The Adverse Childhood Experiences (ACE) Study. *American Journal of Preventive Medicine, 14*(4), 245–258.

Fendrich, M., Weissman, M. M., & Warner, V. (1990). Screening for depressive disorder in children and adolescents: Validating the Center for Epidemiologic Studies Depression Scale for Children. *American Journal of Epidemiology, 131*(3), 538–551.

Forlenza, O. V., De-Paula, V. D. J. R., & Diniz, B. S. O. (2014). Neuroprotective effects of lithium: Implications for the treatment of Alzheimer's disease and related neurodegenerative disorders. *ACS Chemical Neuroscience, 5*(6), 443–450.

Friedrich, M. J. (2017). Depression is the leading cause of disability around the world. *JAMA, 317*(15), 1517.

Gerbarg, P. L. (2019). *Complementary and integrative treatments in psychiatric practice.* Washington, DC: American Psychiatric Association Publishing.

Guaiana, G., & Barbui, C. (2016). Discontinuing benzodiazepines: Best practices. *Epidemiology and Psychiatric Sciences, 25*(3), 214–216.

Guo, T., Xiang, Y. T., Xiao, L., Hu, C. Q., Chiu, H. F., Ungvari, G. S., ... Feng, Y. (2015). Measurement-based care versus standard care for major depression: A randomized controlled trial with blind raters. *American Journal of Psychiatry, 172*(10), 1004–1013.

Guy, W. (1976). *ECDEU assessment manual for psychopharmacology* (Rev. ed.) (DHHS Publication No. ADM 91-338). Washington, DC: U.S. Department of Health, Education, and Welfare.

Hirschfeld, R. M., Williams, J. B., Spitzer, R. L., Calabrese, J. R., Flynn, L., Keck Jr, P. E., ... Russell, J. M. (2000). Development and validation of a screening instrument for bipolar spectrum disorder: The Mood Disorder Questionnaire. *American Journal of Psychiatry, 157*(11), 1873–1875.

Huybrechts, K. F., Hernández-Díaz, S., Patorno, E., Desai, R. J., Mogun, H., Dejene, S. Z., ... Bateman, B. T. (2016). Antipsychotic use in pregnancy and the risk for congenital malformations. *JAMA Psychiatry, 73*(9), 938–946.

James, S. N., Davis, D., O'Hare, C., Sharma, N., John, A., Gaysina, D., ... Richards, M. (2018). Lifetime affective problems and later-life cognitive state: Over 50 years of follow-up in a British birth cohort study. *Journal of Affective Disorders, 241*, 348–355.

Johnson, J. G., Harris, E. S., Spitzer, R. L., & Williams, J. B. (2002). The Patient Health Questionnaire for Adolescents: Validation of an instrument for the assessment of mental disorders among adolescent primary care patients. *Journal of Adolescent Health, 30*(3), 196–204.

Kelly, C. B., McDonnell, A. P., Johnston, T. G., Mulholland, C., Cooper, S. J., McMaster, D., ... Whitehead, A. S. (2004). The MTHFR C677T polymorphism is associated with depressive episodes in patients from Northern Ireland. *Journal of Psychopharmacology, 18*(4), 567–571.

Kroenke, K., Spitzer, R. L., & Williams, J. B. (2001). The PHQ-9: Validity of a brief depression severity measure. *Journal of General Internal Medicine, 16*(9), 606–613.

Lader, M. (2014). Benzodiazepine harm: How can it be reduced? *British Journal of Clinical Pharmacology, 77*(2), 295–301.

Lafeuille, M. H., Dean, J., Carter, V., Duh, M. S., Fastenau, J., Dirani, R., & Lefebvre, P. (2014). Systematic review of long-acting injectables versus oral atypical antipsychotics on hospitalization in schizophrenia. *Current Medical Research and Opinion, 30*(8), 1643–1655.

Lähteenvuo, M., Tanskanen, A., Taipale, H., Hoti, F., Vattulainen, P., Vieta, E., & Tiihonen, J. (2018). Real-world effectiveness of pharmacologic treatments for the prevention of rehospitalization in a Finnish nationwide cohort of patients with bipolar disorder. *JAMA Psychiatry, 75*(4), 347–355.

Lefebvre, P., Muser, E., Joshi, K., DerSarkissian, M., Bhak, R. H., Duh, M. S., ... Young-Xu, Y. (2017). Impact of paliperidone palmitate versus oral atypical antipsychotics on health care resource use and costs in veterans with schizophrenia and comorbid substance abuse. *Clinical Therapeutics, 39*(7), 1380–1395.

Leibenluft, E. (2011). Severe mood dysregulation, irritability, and the diagnostic boundaries of bipolar disorder in youths. *American Journal of Psychiatry, 168*(2), 129–142.

Lewitzka, U., Severus, E., Bauer, R., Ritter, P., Müller-Oerlinghausen, B., & Bauer, M. (2015). The suicide prevention effect of lithium: More than 20 years of evidence—a narrative review. *International Journal of Bipolar Disorders, 3*(1), 15.

Lijster, J. M. D., Dierckx, B., Utens, E. M., Verhulst, F. C., Zieldorff, C., Dieleman, G. C., & Legerstee, J. S. (2017). The age of onset of anxiety disorders: A meta-analysis. *The Canadian Journal of Psychiatry, 62*(4), 237–246.

Lin, L. Y., Sidani, J. E., Shensa, A., Radovic, A., Miller, E., Colditz, J. B., ... Primack, B. A. (2016). Association between social media use and depression among U.S. young adults. *Depression and Anxiety, 33*(4), 323–331.

Machado-Vieira, R., Manji, H. K., & Zarate Jr, C. A. (2009). The role of lithium in the treatment of bipolar disorder: Convergent evidence for neurotrophic effects as a unifying hypothesis. *Bipolar Disorders, 11*, 92–109.

Markota, M., Rummans, T. A., Bostwick, J. M., & Lapid, M. I. (2016). Benzodiazepine use in older adults: Dangers, management, and alternative therapies. *Mayo Clinic Proceedings, 91*(11), 1632–1639.

Marra, E. M., Mazer-Amirshahi, M., Brooks, G., Van Den Anker, J., May, L., & Pines, J. M. (2015). Benzodiazepine prescribing in older adults in U.S. ambulatory clinics and emergency departments (2001–10). *Journal of the American Geriatrics Society, 63*(10), 2074–2081.

Mason, B. J., Quello, S., & Shadan, F. (2018). Gabapentin for the treatment of alcohol use disorder. *Expert Opinion on Investigational Drugs, 27*(1), 113–124.

Mohamed, S., Johnson, G. R., Chen, P., Hicks, P. B., Davis, L. L., Yoon, J., ... Scrymgeour, A. (2017). Effect of antidepressant switching vs. augmentation on remission among patients with major depressive disorder unresponsive to antidepressant treatment: The VAST-D randomized clinical trial. *JAMA, 318*(2), 132–145.

Morken, G., Widen, J. H., & Grawe, R. W. (2008). Non-adherence to antipsychotic medication, relapse and rehospitalization in recent-onset schizophrenia. *BMC Psychiatry, 8*(1), 32.

Morlet, E., Hozer, F., & Costemale-Lacoste, J. F. (2018). Neuroprotective effects of lithium: What are the implications in humans with neurodegenerative disorders? *Geriatrie et Psychologie Neuropsychiatrie du Vieillissement, 16*(1), 78–86.

Morrison, K. E., Cole, A. B., Thompson, S. M., & Bale, T. L. (2019). Brexanolone for the treatment of patients with postpartum depression. *Drugs of Today, 55*(9), 537–544.

Muskin, P. R., Gerbarg, P. L., & Brown, R. P. (2013). Along roads less traveled: Complementary, alternative, and integrative treatments. *Psychiatric Clinics, 36*(1), xiii–xv.

Muzina, D. (2010). Discontinuing an antidepressant? Tapering tips to ease distressing symptoms. *Current Psychiatry, 9*(3), 51–61.

Nikoo, M., Radnia, H., Farokhnia, M., Mohammadi, M. R., & Akhondzadeh, S. (2015). N-acetylcysteine as an adjunctive therapy to risperidone for treatment of irritability in autism: A randomized, double-blind, placebo-controlled clinical trial of efficacy and safety. *Clinical Neuropharmacology, 38*(1), 11–17.

Noordraven, E. L., Wierdsma, A. I., Blanken, P., Bloemendaal, A. F., Staring, A. B., & Mulder, C. L. (2017). Financial incentives for improving adherence to maintenance treatment in patients with psychotic disorders (Money for Medication): A multicentre, open-label, randomized controlled trial. *The Lancet Psychiatry, 4*(3), 199–207.

Noordraven, E. L., Wierdsma, A. I., Blanken, P., Bloemendaal, A. F., & Mulder, C. L. (2018). The effect of financial incentives on patients' motivation for treatment: Results of "Money for Medication," a randomized controlled trial. *BMC Psychiatry, 18*(1), 144.

Nurnberg, H. G., Hensley, P. L., Heiman, J. R., Croft, H. A., Debattista, C., & Paine, S. (2008). Sildenafil treatment of women with antidepressant-associated sexual dysfunction: A randomized controlled trial. *JAMA, 300*(4), 395–404.

Ogbonna, C. I., & Lembke, A. (2017). Tapering patients off of benzodiazepines. *American Family Physician, 96*(9), 606–610.

Pacchiarotti, I., Bond, D. J., Baldessarini, R. J., Nolen, W. A., Grunze, H., Licht, R. W., ... Tondo, L. (2013). The International Society for Bipolar Disorders (ISBD) task force report on antidepressant use in bipolar disorders. *American Journal of Psychiatry, 170*(11), 1249–1262.

Pawełczyk, T., Grancow-Grabka, M., Kotlicka-Antczak, M., Trafalska, E., & Pawełczyk, A. (2016). A randomized controlled study of the efficacy of six-month supplementation with concentrated fish oil rich in omega-3 polyunsaturated fatty acids in first episode schizophrenia. *Journal of Psychiatric Research, 73*, 34–44.

Perlis, M. L., Jungquist, C., Smith, M. T. & Posner, D. (2008). *Cognitive behavioral treatment of insomnia: A session by session guide.* New York: Springer.

Peters, B. R. (2018). *Insomnia solved: A self-directed cognitive behavioral therapy for insomnia (CBTI) program.* Seattle, WA: Author.

Pintor, L., Gastó, C., Navarro, V., Torres, X., & Fañanas, L. (2003). Relapse of major depression after complete and partial remission during a 2-year follow-up. *Journal of Affective Disorders, 73*(3), 237–244.

Pintor, L., Torres, X., Bailles, E., Navarro, V., de Osaba, M. J. M., Belmonte, A., & Gastó, C. (2013). CRF test in melancholic depressive patients with partial versus complete relapses: A 2-year follow-up study. *Nordic Journal of Psychiatry, 67*(3), 177–184.

Post, R. M. (2018). The new news about lithium: An underutilized treatment in the United States. *Neuropsychopharmacology, 43*(5), 1174–1179.

Posternak, M. A., & Mueller, T. I. (2001). Assessing the risks and benefits of benzodiazepines for anxiety disorders in patients with a history of substance abuse or dependence. *American Journal on Addictions, 10*(1), 48–68.

Radovic, A., & Moreno, M. A. (2019). Treatment options for adolescent depression. *JAMA Pediatrics, 173*(3), 300–300.

Rej, S., Beaulieu, S., Segal, M., Low, N. C., Mucsi, I., Holcroft, C., ... Looper, K. J. (2014). Lithium dosing and serum concentrations across the age spectrum: From early adulthood to the tenth decade of life. *Drugs & Aging, 31*(12), 911–916.

Rush, A. J., Trivedi, M. H., Ibrahim, H. M., Carmody, T. J., Arnow, B., Klein, D. N., ... Thase, M. E. (2003). The 16-Item Quick Inventory of Depressive Symptomatology (QIDS), clinician rating (QIDS-C), and self-report (QIDS-SR): A psychometric evaluation in patients with chronic major depression. *Biological Psychiatry, 54*(5), 573–583.

Sareen, J., Cox, B. J., Afifi, T. O., de Graaf, R., Asmundson, G. J., Ten Have, M., & Stein, M. B. (2005). Anxiety disorders and risk for suicidal ideation and suicide attempts: A population-based longitudinal study of adults. *Archives of General Psychiatry, 62*(11), 1249–1257.

Severus, E., Taylor, M. J., Sauer, C., Pfennig, A., Ritter, P., Bauer, M., & Geddes, J. R. (2014). Lithium for prevention of mood episodes in bipolar disorders: Systematic review and meta-analysis. *International Journal of Bipolar Disorders, 2*(1), 15.

Sharma, A., Gerbarg, P., Bottiglieri, T., Massoumi, L., Carpenter, L. L., Lavretsky, H., … Mischoulon, D. (2017). S-Adenosylmethionine (SAMe) for neuropsychiatric disorders: A clinician-oriented review of research. *The Journal of Clinical Psychiatry, 78*(6), e656.

Shear, M. K., Brown, T. A., Barlow, D. H., Money, R., Sholomskas, D. E., Woods, S. W., … Papp, L. A. (1997). Multicenter collaborative Panic Disorder Severity Scale. *American Journal of Psychiatry, 154*(11), 1571–1575.

Shelton, R. C., Pencina, M. J., Barrentine, L. W., Ruiz, J. A., Fava, M., Zajecka, J. M., & Papakostas, G. I. (2015). Association of obesity and inflammatory marker levels on treatment outcome: Results from a double-blind, randomized study of adjunctive L-methylfolate calcium in patients with MDD who are inadequate responders to SSRIs. *The Journal of Clinical Psychiatry, 76*(12), 1635–1641.

Solmi, M., Murru, A., Pacchiarotti, I., Undurraga, J., Veronese, N., Fornaro, M., … & Correll, C. U. (2017). Safety, tolerability, and risks associated with first-and second-generation antipsychotics: A state-of-the-art clinical review. *Therapeutics and Clinical Risk Management, 13*, 757–777.

Somers, J. M., Goldner, E. M., Waraich, P., & Hsu, L. (2006). Prevalence and incidence studies of anxiety disorders: A systematic review of the literature. *The Canadian Journal of Psychiatry, 51*(2), 100–113.

Spitzer, R. L., Kroenke, K., Williams, J. B., & Löwe, B. (2006). A brief measure for assessing generalized anxiety disorder: The GAD-7. *Archives of Internal Medicine, 166*(10), 1092–1097.

Stewart, D. E., & Vigod, S. (2016). Postpartum depression. *New England Journal of Medicine, 375*(22), 2177–2186.

Sujan, A. C., Rickert, M. E., Öberg, A. S., Quinn, P. D., Hernández-Díaz, S., Almqvist, C., … D'Onofrio, B. M. (2017). Associations of maternal antidepressant use during the first trimester of pregnancy with preterm birth, small for gestational age, autism spectrum disorder, and attention-deficit/hyperactivity disorder in offspring. *JAMA, 317*(15), 1553–1562.

Sylvia, L. G., Hay, A., Ostacher, M. J., Miklowitz, D. J., Nierenberg, A. A., Thase, M. E., … Perlis, R. H. (2013). Association between therapeutic alliance, care satisfaction, and pharmacological adherence in bipolar disorder. *Journal of Clinical Psychopharmacology, 33*(3), 343–350.

Tiihonen, J., Tanskanen, A., Hoti, F., Vattulainen, P., Taipale, H., Mehtälä, J., & Lähteenvuo, M. (2017). Pharmacological treatments and risk of readmission to hospital for unipolar depression in Finland: A nationwide cohort study. *The Lancet Psychiatry, 4*(7), 547–553.

Twenge, J. M., Cooper, A. B., Joiner, T. E., Duffy, M. E., & Binau, S. G. (2019). Age, period, and cohort trends in mood disorder indicators and suicide-related outcomes in a nationally representative dataset, 2005–2017. *Journal of Abnormal Psychology, 128*(3), 185–199.

Unützer, J., Katon, W., Callahan, C. M., Williams Jr, J. W., Hunkeler, E., Harpole, L., … Areán, P. A. (2002). Collaborative care management of late-life depression in the primary care setting: A randomized controlled trial. *JAMA, 288*(22), 2836–2845.

Velez-Ruiz, N. J., & Meador, K. J. (2015). Neurodevelopmental effects of fetal antiepileptic drug exposure. *Drug Safety, 38*(3), 271–278.

Viguera, A. C., Whitfield, T., Baldessarini, R. J., Newport, D. J., Stowe, Z., Reminick, A., … Cohen, L. S. (2007). Risk of recurrence in women with bipolar disorder during pregnancy: Prospective study of mood stabilizer discontinuation. *American Journal of Psychiatry, 164*(12), 1817–1824.

Weathers, F. W., Litz, B. T., Keane, T. M., Palmieri, P. A., Marx, B. P., & Schnurr, P. P. (2013). The PTSD Checklist for DSM–5 (PCL-5). Boston, MA: National Center for PTSD.

Wegner, M., Helmich, I., Machado, S. E., Nardi, A., Arias-Carrión, O., & Budde, H. (2014). Effects of exercise on anxiety and depression disorders: Review of meta-analyses and neurobiological mechanisms. *CNS & Neurological Disorders-Drug Targets, 13*(6), 1002–1014.

Wesseloo, R., Wierdsma, A. I., van Kamp, I. L., Munk-Olsen, T., Hoogendijk, W. J., Kushner, S. A., & Berkink, V. (2017). Lithium dosing strategies during pregnancy and the postpartum period. *The British Journal of Psychiatry, 211*(1), 31–36.

Wieck, A. (2017). Prevention of bipolar episodes with lithium in the perinatal period. *The British Journal of Psychiatry, 211*(1), 3–4.

Wink, L. K., Pedapati, E. V., Horn, P. S., McDougle, C. J., & Erickson, C. A. (2017). Multiple antipsychotic medication use in autism spectrum disorder. *Journal of Child and Adolescent Psychopharmacology, 27*(1), 91–94.

World Health Organization. (2017). Depression and common mental disorders: Global health estimates. Geneva: World Health Organization.

Xie, Z., Chen, F., Li, W. A., Geng, X., Li, C., Meng, X., ... Yu, F. (2017). A review of sleep disorders and melatonin. *Neurological Research, 39*(6), 559–565.

Yatham, L. N., Kennedy, S. H., Parikh, S. V., Schaffer, A., Bond, D. J., Frey, B. N., ... Alda, M. (2018). Canadian Network for Mood and Anxiety Treatments (CANMAT) and International Society for Bipolar Disorders (ISBD) 2018 guidelines for the management of patients with bipolar disorder. *Bipolar Disorders, 20*(2), 97–170.

Yesavage, J. A., Brink, T. L., Rose, T. L., Lum, O., Huang, V., Adey, M., & Leirer, V. O. (1982). Development and validation of a geriatric depression screening scale: A preliminary report. *Journal of Psychiatric Research, 17*(1), 37–49.

Zhou, X., Ravindran, A. V., Qin, B., Del, C. G., Li, Q., Bauer, M., ... Wang, X. (2015). Comparative efficacy, acceptability, and tolerability of augmentation agents in treatment-resistant depression: Systematic review and network meta-analysis. *The Journal of Clinical Psychiatry, 76*(4), e487–498.